Wall Pilates Worko
Women

Transform Your Body in Minutes a Day with 90+ Illustrated Exercises for Strength, Flexibility, and Total Body Toning 9 Bonus Inside

Daisy Cote

Wall Pilates Workouts for Women

© Copyright 2024 by Daisy Cote
All rights reserved

TABLE OF CONTENTS

Daisy Cote

INTRODUCTION

The Philosophy Behind Wall Pilates

Wall Pilates focuses on building core strength and overall tone using the support of a wall to stabilize the body during standing exercises. This form of Pilates is based on the teachings of Joseph Pilates, a German physical trainer, writer and inventor who developed a system of total body conditioning in the early 20th century.

The philosophy behind Wall Pilates is to engage the deep stabilizing muscles along the center of the body known as the "powerhouse" through controlled movements. This strengthens the abdominals, back muscles, pelvic floor and shoulders to improve posture, balance, stability and quality of movement. Performing Pilates with a wall as a prop allows people to perform exercises safely with proper alignment while reaping the full benefits of traditional mat Pilates. Joseph Pilates emphasized activating the mind-body connection using breath with movement, controlling the body precisely and improving flexibility as well as strength. Wall Pilates incorporates all of these core principles. By stabilizing against the wall, people can maintain proper alignment as they engage their core and concentrate on smooth, flowing motions. The wall provides feedback and assists with balance while ensuring the deep muscles must work to stabilize the joints. This allows for a full range of motion within safe limits.

Wall Pilates is extremely versatile and can be modified for all fitness levels. Beginners can start with basic moves to develop core awareness and control. Intermediate and advanced students can add resistance or challenges to progress. Since exercises are done standing or seated, because of how gentle it is on the joints. The wall provides assistance for those with limitations, injuries or aching muscles. Pilates marries physical and mental discipline, making practitioners more mindful, centered and in tune with their bodies.

Wall Pilates requires no equipment other than a wall as the name implies, making it accessible and convenient to perform anytime and anywhere. The exercises build functional fitness that translates directly into everyday living. A stronger core lends power to regular activities and sports while improved balance and alignment prevents injuries and facilitate natural, graceful movements. Pilates enhances physical and mental well-being, allowing people to move with purpose, precision and poise.

Wall Pilates offers a time-efficient way to condition the entire body. Just 10-30 minutes a day can sculpt a strong core and toned physique. The wall provides stability for beginners, but also resistance to amplify the challenge. Controlled movements concentrate effort in the core muscles while working upper and lower body simultaneously in one integrated system. Practicing Wall Pilates consistently will transform strength, flexibility, and form.

With its emphasis on precise movements coordinated with breath, Pilates exemplifies the mind-body connection. The core principles strengthen physical control and awareness in equal measure. Using the wall as a training tool allows optimal alignment and safety during standing exercises. Wall Pilates builds full-body fitness and balances all muscle groups in harmonious motion. The benefits extend beyond the physical, to focus the mind, decompress stress and promote overall wellness.

CHAPTER 1

GETTING STARTED WITH WALL PILATES

The Basics of Wall Pilates

Wall Pilates utilizes the support of a wall to assist, strengthen and challenge the body during standing or seated exercises. This allows for proper alignment, body awareness and core engagement while performing movements adapted from mat Pilates. Wall Pilates provides an excellent introduction to the Pilates method and its benefits. Even seasoned practitioners continue to incorporate the wall into their routines for optimal posture, safety and control.

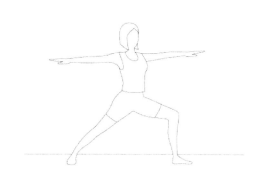

The most basic principle of any Pilates practice is breath and core control. All exercises begin with proper breathing, pulling the navel to spine to activate the deep abdominals and pelvic floor. While doing this, it is important that the core remains engaged throughout movements. The wall plays its part by providing feedback and cues to maintain the upright, neutral alignment of the spine. While doing this, the shoulders need to stay down and rested back to keep the chest open.

Wall Pilates movements are small and precise, it focuses more on quality and not quantity. Each exercise consists of smooth, controlled motions coordinated with breathing while the wall provides an assist with balance and stability so beginners can master the proper form. Going through the full range of motion with control, builds core strength, increasing flexibility with flowing motions.

Essential Equipment and Setup

One of the benefits of Wall Pilates is that it requires minimal equipment. All that is needed to start practicing is a wall, your body, and the commitment to better your health. However, there are a few key pieces of gear that can enhance your Wall Pilates experience and progress. Thoughtfully equipping your workout space will set you up for comfort, safety and success.

Your Wall Pilates space should allow ample room to stand at least one arm's length from the wall. Make sure the area is clear of furniture or clutter. Choose a wall with a flat, smooth surface, a painted or varnished drywall would be ideal. But if it happens to be a textured wall, it can be covered with a cork or foam mats to enable grip and protect the hands. For standing exercises, wear comfortable exercise clothes that give room for flexibility. Tight-fitting garments allow you to check alignment and bare feet or grip socks enable traction. While workout shoes are not required, cross trainers provide arch support if exercises are performed standing. It's important to avoid slippery socks or bulky shoes.

Mats also provide cushioning and traction if performing floor work, a standard Pilates mat around 5 millimeters thick is sufficient. For knee comfort, a foldable exercise mat can be layered on top. Yoga mats also work if the mat is thicker than typical Pilates mats. Another essential thing to do is to position the mats perpendicular to the wall during standing exercises.

Resistance bands add intensity when looped around the legs, arms or shoulders. Starting with light resistance bands and progressing gradually as strength increases is advisable. Mini looped bands are mostly convenient and easily fit in a pocket, however, longer flat bands allow more versatility. The quality of the rubber needs to also be put into consideration as it has to be of high quality and needs to be replaced as soon as it starts showing signs of getting worn out. Specific Pilates equipment like a magic circle or Pilates ring boosts resistance for both arms and legs while the versatile ring tones the entire body. Foam rollers assist in spinal articulation and stretching, weighted balls target core strength when held during exercises while ankle and wrist weights increase lower and upper body intensity.

Small Pilates balls on the other hand, allow seated exercises. The peanut-shaped balls fit between the knees or inner thighs for adductor work and the much larger inflated balls act as cushions and props for balance challenges. These balls need to be deflated when they are not being used to maintain their shapes properly. They also need to be checked for leaks, tears or defects regularly. For easy workouts anytime, a Pilates Power Gym spring attachment can be used on any door. It lets you do standing Pilates moves. You can also use arm and leg straps with door anchors for resistance in different directions. Begin with lighter resistance bands and move up as you get stronger. Make sure to install and check the attachments properly.

While all you need for Wall Pilates is a wall, adding a few key props can enhance your routine; Things like bands, balls and Pilates equipment such as rings can add variety and help you progress. It's important to pick equipment that's well-made, adaptable and suitable for your skill level. Take care of your equipment to make sure it lasts. If you don't have certain equipment, you can still modify exercises to work without it. By thoughtfully incorporating props, you can take your Wall Pilates workout to the next level.

Above all, listen to your body and work within your limits using modifications as needed. Proper form and awareness should be prioritized rather than straining with added resistance. Respect pain signals immediately and adjust intensity accordingly. Appropriately leveled equipment will provide a safe and effective workout. With mindful attention and optimal setup, a wall and your own body weight can provide an incredibly effective Pilates routine. Adding equipment introduces creativity, variety and increased intensity over time.

Get ready for a great Wall Pilates session by setting up your space, getting quality gear and keeping a beginner's mindset focused on precision and not intensity. Pay attention to proper form and have a compassionate approach with your exercise. That's the recipe for a phenomenal Wall Pilates experience.

Safety Measures and Injury Prevention

Wall Pilates provides an excellent way to develop core strength, flexibility and balance with the assistance of a wall for support. However, as with any physical fitness routine, proper form and reasonable precautions are necessary to avoid strain or injury. Approaching Wall Pilates with mindfulness, listening to your body, and gradually advancing through the difficulty will keep your practice safe while still offering incredible benefits.

When it comes to staying safe during any workout, remember the basics of injury prevention. Start by warming up properly before you exercise and cooling down afterwards. Stretching cold muscles too quickly can lead to tears and pulls, so take your time. Try dynamic warm-ups to get your blood flowing and increase your range of motion. After your workout, cool down gradually to avoid feeling dizzy or straining your muscles. Remember to stay hydrated, eat well and give your body time to rest between intense workouts.

When first adopting Wall Pilates, begin slowly especially if new to fitness. Attempting overly advanced exercises without proper preparation risks muscle or joint problems. Build a foundation first focusing on posture, alignment, gentle stretches and breath control. Master the basic movements before going for the complex ones. Stick to movements that match your current mobility and stability levels and void pushing yourself too far or sacrificing proper form. It's okay to make modifications, like bending your knees, limiting your range of motion, using support, or lowering resistance. The key is to work within your capabilities to stay safe and prevent injuries. There is no shame in simplifying exercises to respect your body's limits. The idea is to make progress at an appropriate pace without expectation.

Focus on maintaining correct alignment and technique throughout every exercise. Keep your shoulders relaxed, engage your core to support your spine and keep your pelvis in a neutral position. It's more important to maintain good form than to push through sloppy movements. If you feel any sharp pain during any exercise, stop immediately and reassess your positioning. Adjust as many times as may be needed to prevent injury, try to avoid jerky, momentum-driven motions. Pilates focuses on smooth, controlled movements coordinated with breathing. Moving too quickly, hinging or twisting while carrying weight increases the risk of acute muscle tears or ligament sprains. It's just as risky to stretch too far without warming up properly. Always ease into flexibility exercises after warming up to avoid injury.

Check the stability and traction of the wall and floor at all times when exercising. Textured surfaces generally provide more grip so ensure that there's no risk of slipping or sliding during any of the exercises. Declutter workout areas, watch for trip hazards and make use of mats, shoes or socks to increase traction as needed. It is important to include rest days in your workout routine to avoid overtraining. Muscles need time to recover and strengthen. Mix high-intensity exercises with gentle stretching and breath work to keep your body balanced. Rotate through different muscle groups and ranges of motion to prevent overuse.

Listen to your body's signals carefully, pain is usually a sign that something's wrong somewhere and needs attention. Joint, tendon and ligament pain could indicate problems with your technique. It's better to ease off or modify your workout than to push through real pain. Taking care of your body now will help keep you healthy in the long run.

Be kind to yourself when you make mistakes or face limitations. Progress isn't always smooth, it's normal to have good and bad days. Expect setbacks and times when you may feel stuck, but also celebrate your small victories every day. With patience and consistency, you'll make remarkable progress. Enjoy the process!

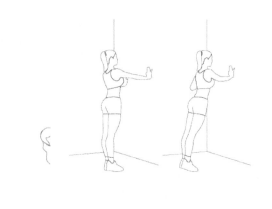

Pre-Workout Warm-Up Routines

For a focused routine such as Wall Pilates which emphasizes strength, flexibility and total body toning, incorporating a targeted pre-workout warm-up is essential. These warm-up exercises are designed to prepare your muscles and joints for the specific demands of Wall Pilates, enhancing both the effectiveness and safety of your workout.

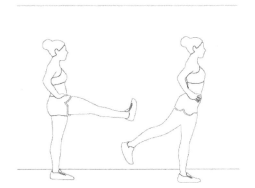

1. Wall Push-Aways

How to Do It:

- Stand facing a wall, about an arm's length away.

- Place your palms flat against the wall at shoulder height.

- Lean your body towards the wall, bending your elbows then push your body back to the starting position using your arm strength.

Duration: 10-12 repetitions.

Benefits: Warms up the shoulders, chest and arms while activating core stability, preparing the upper body for exercises that require pushing or arm stability.

2. Wall-Assisted Leg Swings

How to Do It:

- Stand sideways next to the wall, lightly holding it for balance.

- Swing the leg closest to the wall back and forth in a controlled manner, keeping your torso upright.

- Perform the swings on one leg, then turn around to repeat with the other leg.

Duration: 10-15 swings per leg.

Benefits: Increases hip mobility and warms up the leg muscles, preparing for movements that involve leg extensions and lifts in Pilates.

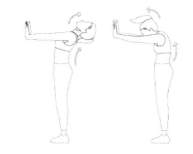

3. Wall Slides

How to Do It:

- Stand with your back against a wall, feet about hip-width apart.

- Slide down into a squat position, keeping your back flat against the wall.

- Slide back up to the starting position.

Duration: 10-12 repetitions.

Benefits: Activates the lower body, particularly the quadriceps, hamstrings and glutes. It also helps to improve the range of motion in the knees and hips.

4. Wall-Assisted Cat-Cow Stretch

How to Do It:
- Place your hands on the wall at waist height.

- Arch your back and tilt your head upwards as you inhale (Cow).

- Round your spine and tuck your chin to your chest as you exhale (Cat).

Duration: 8-10 slow and controlled repetitions.

Benefits: Enhances spinal flexibility and warms up the back muscles, crucial for maintaining proper posture and alignment in Pilates exercises.

5. Wall Toe

How to Do It:

- Stand facing the wall with your arms extended for balance.

- Lift one foot and tap the wall with your toes, then alternate with the other foot.

- Duration: 15-20 taps per foot.

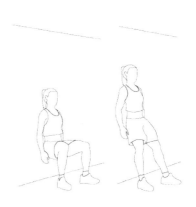

Benefits: Warms up the calves and ankles, promoting balance and stability, which are essential for performing Pilates movements that require precise control and coordination.

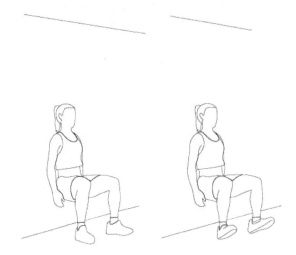

CHAPTER 2

CORE FUNDAMENTALS

Anatomy of the Core

The "core" refers to the muscles that stabilize, align and move the trunk of the body. Core strength is essential for posture, balance and efficient movement. Pilates emphasizes building a strong, responsive core through targeted exercises. Understanding core anatomy allows you to engage the proper muscles during Wall Pilates. The core includes all muscles of the abdomen, lower back, hips and pelvic floor. The rectus abdominis, nicknamed the "six-pack" muscle, flexes the spine to lift the torso. Obliques on the side, bend and rotate the waist. The transverse abdominis wraps around the midsection like a corset, squeezing inward during exhalation.

The erector spinae muscles run vertically to extend the spine while the quadratus lumborum muscles in the low back help the sides bend. Hip flexors, glutes and thighs also provide stability around the core. Meanwhile, the pelvic floor at the base of the abdomen supports internal organs.

Proper core activation begins with breath. Inhaling causes diaphragm contraction, pressurizing the abdomen while exhaling draws the navel in towards the spine, engaging deep abdominals. Pilates emphasizes lateral thoracic breathing, maximizing oxygenation. Proper spinal alignment is crucial during core exercises. When excercising, maintain the spine's natural curves, with a slight arch in the neck and low back, while keeping the mid-back and sacrum neutral. Engage your abdominals to prevent overarching. Additionally, ensure your shoulder blades are pinched together and downward. During Wall Pilates, the core stabilizes the body against gravity. Isometric holds challenge endurance and controlled motions test coordination. Using the wall gives you instant feedback on your posture and over time, you'll get better at engaging your core muscles during everyday activities.

Here's an example: when doing shoulder presses against the wall, make sure to keep your spine straight as you press your palms back into the wall. Avoid leaning forward or arching your back too much. As you exhale, tighten your abs to keep your spine aligned. Your obliques will help stabilize your torso when doing side presses. When practicing spinal articulation, it's important to focus on isolating each curve of the spine instead of slouching through the back. Start by rounding your shoulders forward and drawing your navel in to flex the upper spine. Then, tilt your pelvis back to extend the lower spine while making sure not to flare your ribs or overarch your back.

During leg lowers, keep the core engaged to stabilize the pelvis. Don't let the back sag as legs lift parallel to the floor. Use the wall for balance, relying on abdominals rather than momentum to control the movement. Mastering proper core activation takes practice but improvements can be noticed over time. Additionally, core exercises can be progressed by using resistance bands or light weights. When you feel prepared, gradually move away from the wall to increase the demands on your balance and strength. Focus on maintaining precision and control as you progress, being mindful not to compensate through othermuscles. Increase the number of repetitions or duration gradually while ensuring proper form is maintained throughout. A strong, responsive core transforms posture, balance and coordination. Pilates builds functional fitness utilizing movements drawn from daily life. The core integrates the entire body into a stable, mobile system. Cultivating awareness and control helps unlock this incredible potential within.

Beginner Exercises

1. Wall Mountain Climbers

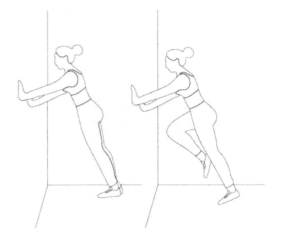

How to Do It:

- Start by facing the wall, placing your hands on the wall at about chest level, slightly wider than shoulder-width apart.

- Step back so your body forms a diagonal line from your head to your heels, similar to a push-up position against the wall.

- Engage your core and lift one knee towards the wall, then return it and switch to the other knee.

- Continue alternating knees with a focus on keeping your hips stable and your core engaged throughout the movement.

Duration: Begin with 2 sets of 10 repetitions per leg, gradually increasing as you build endurance and strength.

Benefits: This exercise not only activates the core muscles but also involves the shoulders and lower body, providing a comprehensive workout that enhances core stability and coordination.

2. Wall Plank

How to Do It:

- Face the wall and place your forearms on the wall at shoulder height, keeping your elbows under your shoulders.

- Step back until your body is in a straight line from your head to your heels, similar to a plank position on the floor but elevated against the wall.

- Engage your core, squeeze your glutes and hold this position. Ensure your back remains flat and your hips don't sag or pike up.

Duration: Start by holding the position for 20-30 seconds, gradually increasing the duration as your core strength improves.

Benefits: The wall plank is excellent for beginners as it reduces the strain on the lower back while still effectively engaging the entire core. This position also helps in building endurance and stability in the core muscles, which is fundamental for progressing to more advanced Pilates exercises.

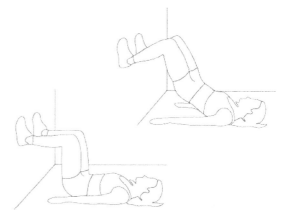

Intermediate Exercises

1. Wall Bridges

How to Do It:

- Lie on your back with your feet flat against the wall, knees bent at a 90-degree angle.

- Place your arms flat at your sides for stability.

- Press your feet into the wall as you lift your hips off the floor, aiming to create a straight line from your shoulders to your knees.

- Hold at the top for a few seconds then slowly lower your hips back to the starting position.

Duration: Perform 2-3 sets of 12-15 repetitions.

Benefits: Wall Bridges primarily target the core and lower back but also engage the glutes and hamstrings. This exercise enhances pelvic stability and strengthens the lower back, which is crucial for overall core performance in more advanced Pilates exercises.

2. Wall Oblique Twists

How to Do It:

- Stand about 2 feet away from the wall, facing sideways.

- Keep your feet firmly planted and hold a lightweight medicine ball or a similar weighted object at chest level.

- Twist your torso to face the wall and gently throw the ball against the wall.

- Catch the ball on the rebound, twist back to the starting position and repeat.

- After completing the set, switch sides to ensure both sides of the obliques are worked equally.

Duration: Perform 2 sets of 10-12 repetitions on each side.

Benefits: This exercise focuses on the obliques, enhancing rotational strength and flexibility. It's excellent for building a more responsive and resilient core, which improves balance, coordination, and overall functional fitness.

Advanced Exercises

1. Wall V-Sits

How to Do It:

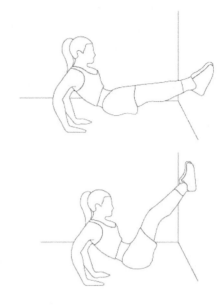

- Sit on the floor facing away from the wall with your legs extended straight in front of you.

- Place your hands on the floor behind you for support and place your heels against the bottom of the wall.

- Lean back slightly and lift your legs, pressing your heels against the wall so your body forms a V-shape.

- Hold this position, engaging your core to maintain balance and stability.

- For added intensity, extend your arms forward, parallel to the ground.

Duration: Hold the V-sit for 20-30 seconds, performing 3-4 sets.

Benefits: This exercise intensely targets the core muscles, including the rectus abdominis and the obliques. It improves balance, enhances core endurance and increases overall abdominal strength.

2. Wall Leg Raises with a Twist

How to Do It:

- Lie on your back on the floor with your head away from the wall and your legs extended upwards against the wall.

- Keep your lower back pressed into the floor and place your hands flat beside you for stability.

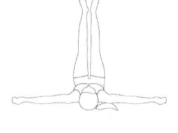

- Lower your legs down towards the floor in a controlled manner then lift them back up to the wall.

- Add a twist by rotating your legs slightly to each side alternately when they are lowered to engage the obliques.

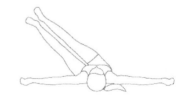

Duration: Perform 10-12 repetitions per side for 2-3 sets.

Benefits: This exercise enhances control and strength in the lower abs and obliques. The leg raise works the deep core muscles, while the added twist increases the challenge and effectiveness for the obliques, aiding in better rotational movement and lateral strength.

CHAPTER 3

UPPER BODY FOCUS

Benefits of Upper Body Strength

Many only associate Pilates with core strength but the method also builds incredible upper body capabilities. The arms bear weight in daily life - pushing, pulling, lifting and stabilizing. Wall Pilates exercises target the shoulders, chest, back and arms, improving function and preventing injury. Developing upper body control and endurance enables activities of daily living with ease and confidence. The shoulder girdle provides incredible mobility at the expense of stability. Various small muscles coordinate complex shoulder movements. Wall Pilates arm exercises reinforce shoulder integration and alignment. Pressing into the wall engages scapular muscles to stabilize the shoulders. Arm circles and swings increase the range of motion. Over time, activities like reaching overhead or behind the back become more comfortable.

Pushing and pressing movements also build upper body endurance. Shoulder taps, planks and side arm raises strengthen the arms both isometrically and dynamically. Integrating breath control to exertion helps improve conditioning even more. Changing the hand position—whether it's wide, narrow, high, or low— challenges the muscles in different ways. Gradually increasing the number of repetitions or the duration of exercises will lead to noticeable improvements in upper body fitness. Many daily tasks require pulling strength as well - opening doors, carrying bags and lifting children. Wall Pilates rowing movements target back muscles like the lats and rhomboids. Scapular retraction and depression during rows improves posture.

Resistance bands add intensity to these rows at various angles for a more complete upper back workout. The chest and arms also benefit from Wall Pilates routines. Modified pushups on the wall reinforce the challenging plank position safely, while triceps dips and bicep curls can be integrated into standing or seated flows. When ready, increase the difficulty by adding light hand weights. The key is to focus on the mind-muscle connection, which helps isolate specific muscle groups. Rotator cuff and posterior deltoid muscles help stabilize and mobilize the shoulders. External rotation, internal rotation and abduction when done carefully, canstrengthen these important yet underworked muscles and when balanced with pressing moves, improves shoulder health and overall function.

Wall arm exercises quickly build visible definition in the arms, shoulders and upper back. These benefits however, extend way beyond aesthetics; Improved posture minimizes hunching and strains associated with desk work or driving, healthy shoulders and upper body mechanics make activities like yard work, cleaning, sports or playing with kids much easier on the body. The greatest benefits of upper body Wall Pilates stem from real- world functionality. Controlled strength training translates to lifting heavy items properly – with the legs, not straining the back. Arms and shoulders integration give confidence in balance during activities like yoga, dancing, hiking or even getting up from a fall. Pilates focuses on achieving overall, well-rounded strength training. The core is crucial for providing central stability, while strong arms and shoulders enhance mobility. Unlike mat routines, Standing Wall Pilates lets you condition both your upper and lower body at the same time. Make sure to evenly integrate exercises for the biceps, triceps, chest, back and shoulders to get the best results.

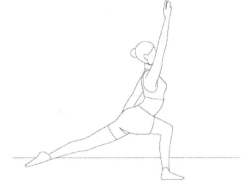

With consistency, Wall Pilates reshapes the upper body. Muscular endurance will increase, allowing longer durations in plank or side planks. Shoulder flexibility will improve through full articulation. Overall posture and carriage will transform as the back strengthens. Soon you'll notice everyday activities that were once difficult, will become fluid and painless. So don't underestimate the upper body aspects of Pilates. The coordinated strength develops through intentional, controlled movements. Patience allows steady gains over time. With full commitment, Wall Pilates can completely transform the shoulders, arms and back for life.

Beginner Upper Body Exercises

1. Wall Push-Ups

How to Do It:

- Stand facing the wall at arm's length, place your hands on the wall slightly wider than shoulder-width apart.

- Keep your feet together and body in a straight line then bend your elbows to lower your chest towards the wall.

- Push back to the starting position and keep your body straight throughout the movement.

Duration: Perform 2-3 sets of 10-15 repetitions.

Benefits: Wall push-ups are a great way to build strength in the chest, shoulders and triceps without the intensity of full floor push-ups, making them suitable for beginners.

2. Wall Slides

How to Do It:

- Stand with your back against the wall and place your arms against the wall with elbows bent at 90 degrees (like a goalpost).

- Slowly slide your arms upwards, keeping them pressed against the wall then slide them back down to the starting position.

Duration: Perform 2-3 sets of 10-12 repetitions.

Benefits: This exercise helps increase shoulder mobility and strengthens the upper back and shoulder muscles.

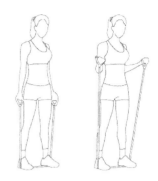

3. Wall Bicep Curls

How to Do It:

- Stand facing the wall with your elbow and forearm pressed against the wall, palm facing upward, holding a light resistance band under your foot.

- Curl your hand towards your shoulder, keeping your forearm pressed against the wall.

- Slowly lower back down.

Duration: Perform 2-3 sets of 10-15 repetitions on each arm.

Benefits: Isolates the biceps effectively, ensuring proper form and enhancing muscle tone without needing heavy weights.

4. Wall Angels

How to Do It:

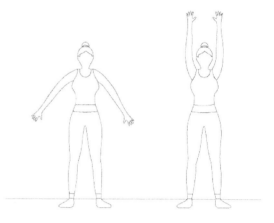

- Stand with your back against the wall, feet about 4 inches from the wall. Keep your back and head touching the wall.

- Extend your arms out to the sides with elbows bent and palms facing forward, then slide your arms up over your head and back down, maintaining contact with the wall.

Duration: Perform 2-3 sets of 10-15 repetitions.

Benefits: Improves posture and shoulder flexibility while strengthening the upper back and shoulder muscles.

5. Wall Chest Squeeze

How to Do It:

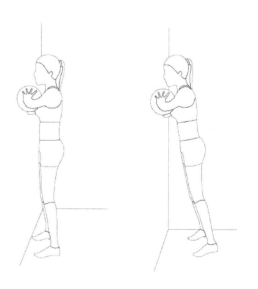

- Stand facing the wall, place a soft ball or Pilates ring between your palms at chest height.

- Press into the ball or ring with both hands, squeeze and hold for a few seconds, then release.

Duration: Perform 2-3 sets of 10-12 squeezes.

Benefits: This exercise targets the chest and front shoulders, helping to build strength and endurance in the pectoral muscles.

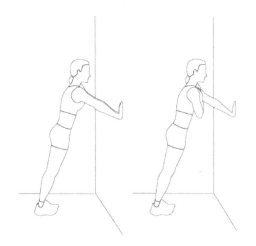

Intermediate Upper Body Exercises

1. Wall Plank Shoulder Taps

How to Do It:

- Start in a plank position with your feet against the wall and hands on the ground directly under your shoulders.

- Lift one hand and tap the opposite shoulder then switch hands, all while keeping your hips steady and not letting them sway.

Duration: Perform 2-3 sets of 10 taps per shoulder.

Benefits: This exercise strengthens the shoulders, chest and core while improving balance and stability.

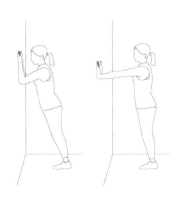

2. Wall Tricep Dips

How to Do It:

- Sit with your back to the wall, legs extended forward and palms on the floor behind you, fingers pointing towards your back.

- Press your palms into the floor and lift your body, sliding your back along the wall.

- Lower your body by bending your elbows until they are at about a 90-degree angle then press back up.

Duration: 2-3 sets of 8-12 repetitions.

Benefits: Targets the triceps, shoulders and upper back, enhancing arm strength and muscle tone.

3. Incline Wall Push-Ups

How to Do It:

- Place your hands on the wall at chest height, slightly wider than shoulder-width.

- Step your feet back so your body is at an inclined angle.

- Perform a push-up, bending your elbows and lowering your chest to the wall then push back to start.

Duration: 2-3 sets of 10-15 repetitions.

Benefits: Increases the difficulty of traditional wall push-ups, targeting the chest, shoulders and core more intensely.

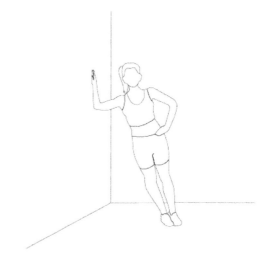

4. Wall Side Plank

How to Do It:

- Start with your side to the wall, place your closest hand on the floor and lean your feet against the wall.

- Lift your body up into a side plank position, keeping your free hand on your hip or extending it upwards.

Duration: Hold for 20-30 seconds on each side, performing 2 3 sets.

Benefits: Strengthens the obliques and shoulders, improves balance and core stability.

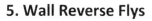
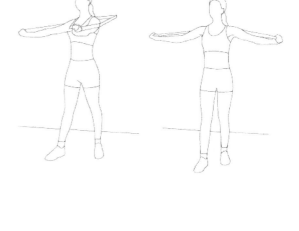

5. Wall Reverse Flys

How to Do It:

- Stand facing the wall, a few feet away, holding a resistance band with both hands, anchored at a point on the wall.

- Extend your arms forward then pull them back and out to the sides, squeezing your shoulder blades together.

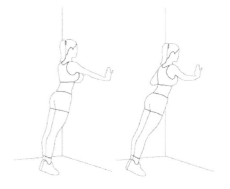

Duration: 2-3 sets of 10-12 repetitions.

Benefits: This exercise targets the rear deltoids and upper back, improving posture and shoulder stability.

6. Wall Mounted Pike Press

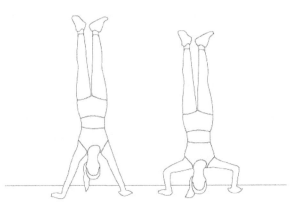

How to Do It:

- Start in a handstand position with your feet against the wall and hands on the floor.
- Bend at the elbows to lower your head towards the ground in a controlled pike press, then push back up.

Duration: 2-3 sets of 6-8 repetitions.

Benefits: Advanced exercise that targets the shoulders, upper chest, and triceps while also engaging the core.

Advanced Upper Body Exercises

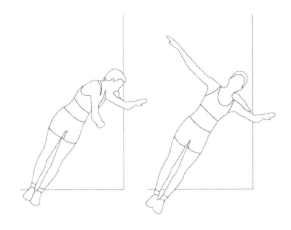

1. Elevated Wall Handstand Push-Ups

How to Do It:

- Begin in a handstand position with your feet resting against the wall and hands placed on the floor shoulder-width apart.
- Lower your body by bending your elbows until your head nearly touches the floor then push back up to the starting position.

Duration: 2-3 sets of 5-8 repetitions.

Benefits: Targets the shoulders, triceps and upper chest and greatly enhances upper body strength and balance.

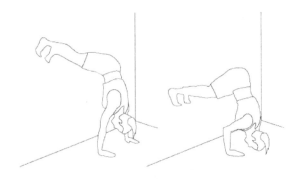

2. Wall Plank Rotations

How to Do It:

- Start in a plank position with your feet against the wall.
- Rotate your body to one side into a side plank

while extending the top arm towards the ceiling.

- Return to the plank position then rotate to the other side.

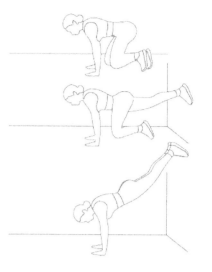

Duration: 2-3 sets of 8-10 rotations per side.

Benefits: Strengthens the core, shoulders and obliques, improving rotational strength and stability.

3. One-Arm Wall Push

How to Do It:

- Stand facing the wall, place one hand in the center of the wall.

- Push off the wall using only one arm, trying to extend fully then slowly return to the starting position.

Duration: 2-3 sets of 10-12 pushes per arm.

Benefits: Enhances unilateral upper body strength, focusing on the chest, shoulders and triceps.

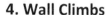

4. Wall Climbs

How to Do It:

- Start in a plank position with your feet against the wall.

- Walk your feet up the wall while walking your hands backward towards the wall, climbing as high as you can.

- Walk back down to the starting position.

Duration: 2-3 sets of 3-5 climbs.

Benefits: Builds full-body strength and control, with a significant focus on the upper body and core.

5. Inverted Wall Rows

How to Do It:

- Begin in an inverted position with your back to the wall, holding a pair of resistance bands attached to the bottom of the wall.

- Pull your chest up towards the bands while

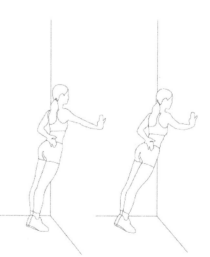

squeezing your shoulder blades together.

Duration: 2-3 sets of 8-10 repetitions.

Benefits: Focuses on the upper back and biceps, improving posture and back strength.

6. Dynamic Wall Chest Flies

How to Do It:

- Stand facing away from the wall in a staggered stance then hold a resistance band in each hand, with bands anchored to a point behind you on the wall.

- Extend your arms out to the sides then dynamically bring them together in front of your chest, and then back out to the sides.

Duration: 2-3 sets of 10-12 repetitions.

Benefits: Works the chest and front deltoids, enhancing muscle tone and endurance.

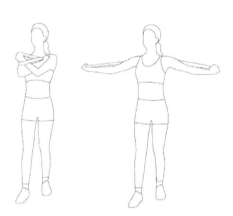

CHAPTER 4

LOWER BODY AND GLUTES ENHANCEMENT

Importance of Lower Body Strength

Lower body strength provides the foundation for mobility, balance and injury prevention. The muscles of the hips, thighs and calves work cohesively during standing, walking and more strenuous activities. Pilates emphasizes full-body conditioning, utilizing the wall to integrate lower and upper body strengthening safely. Improving control and stamina in your legs enhances functional fitness. The gluteal muscles are key; they drive movement by extending the hips and thighs. Wall squats are great for progressively challenging the glutes, starting from partial range of motion and working up to full depth. Engaging your glutes also helps stabilize your pelvis and prevent strain on your back. For dynamic targeting of the glutes, bridging motions are super effective. The quadriceps, located on the front of the thighs, are responsible for straightening and lifting the legs, wall sits are excellent for holding the thighs parallel, which builds endurance in the quads isometrically. Knee lifts and knee tucks engage the quads concentrically, helping to flex the knee joint. When targeting the posterior chain, including the hamstrings, try hamstring curls on the wall.

The inner thighs house the hip adductor muscles, which pull the legs together. You can train these muscles with small pulses. The piriformis muscles, on the other hand, laterally rotate the legs and stretch the hips. To strengthen the lower leg, including the gastrocnemius and soleus muscles, try calf raises. Don't forget about ankle mobility, practicing movements like inversion, eversion and flexion helps maintain full articulation in the ankles. Proper alignment is crucial when conditioning the legs. Keep your knees aligned over your ankles and engage your thighs and glutes without locking your joints. Make sure to maintain a neutral pelvis and spine as you move through your full range of motion. Stack your ankles, knees and hips to integrate your limbs effectively. Exercises such as squats and lunges are functional moves that translate to real life activities like sitting into a chair, getting up from the floor or climbing stairs. These basic daily activities engage the same muscles and patterns. With Wall Pilates, you can master these exercises with the support of the wall before advancing to performing them freestanding.

Like any strength training, it's important to balance progressive overload with adequate recovery. Gradually increase the number of reps or sets within your capabilities. Keep challenging your muscles by varying foot positions or range of motion. Give your muscles at least 48 hours of rest between strength sessions to allow them to rebuild and recover from micro tears.

Beyond muscle definition or aesthetics, lower body Pilates develops key physical competencies for daily life activities. Leg strength improves gait and balance, preventing falls, stability enables activities like carrying heavy loads up a flight of stairs or lifting objects over the head. Knee and ankle control also boost athletics performance while reducing the risk of having an injury. While pelvic and hip flexibility creates better comfort when sitting or driving for a long period of time.

The importance of regular training cannot be more emphasized as regular training also leads to improvements in posture. Activating the glutes and thighs helps untilt the pelvis from an anterior tilt. Aim to keep your shoulders balanced directly over your hips for optimal spinal alignment when exercising. Additionally, regularly stretching your hip flexors helps keep these muscles long and mobile, further enhancing your posture. While lower body strength forms the base, integration with the upper body truly elevates Pilates benefits. Total body conditioning promotes coordinated movement patterns that mirror real-life demands. Wall exercises enable dynamic transitions between arm and leg movements, replicating real-world motions. To achieve balanced fitness, train complementary muscle groups simultaneously, ensuring comprehensive development. With dedication, Pilates done correctly will reshape the lower body remarkably. Consistency and commitment are also key, allowing gradual gains over time and integrating wise progression, ample recovery and optimal nutrition will yield noticeable and incredible improvements in posture, ease of movement and functionality. The entirety of the journey brings empowerment.

Beginner Lower Body Exercises

1. Wall Squats

How to Do It:

- Stand with your back against the wall, feet shoulder-width apart and about two feet from the wall.

- Slide down the wall into a squat position until your thighs are parallel to the floor, keeping your back flat against the wall.

- Hold the position, then slide back up.

Duration: 2-3 sets of 8-10 repetitions.

Benefits: Strengthens the quadriceps, hamstrings, and glutes, and helps build stability and endurance.

2. Wall Assisted Lunges

How to Do It:

- Stand facing away from the wall then step forward with one foot and lean back slightly so your back foot's toes rest against the wall.

- Lower into a lunge, keeping your front knee aligned

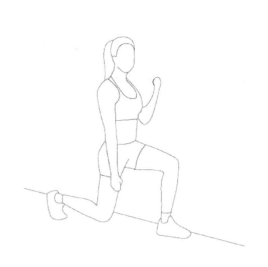

with your ankle.

- Push back up to the starting position.

Duration: 2-3 sets of 8-10 repetitions on each leg.

Benefits: Targets the glutes and thighs, improves balance and coordination.

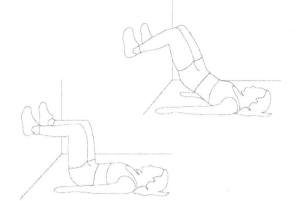

3. Wall Glute Bridges

How to Do It:

- Lie on your back with your feet flat against the wall and knees bent.

- Lift your hips towards the ceiling, squeezing your glutes at the top of the movement.

- Lower your hips back down without touching the floor and repeat.

Duration: 2-3 sets of 10-12 repetitions.

Benefits: Strengthens the glutes, hamstrings and lower back, enhancing pelvic stability and lower body strength.

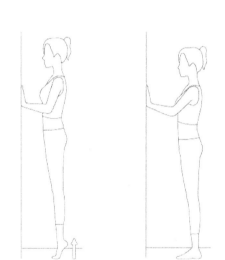

4. Wall Calf Raises

How to Do It:

- Stand facing the wall at arm's length and place your hands on the wall for balance.

- Lift your heels off the ground, rising onto your toes then slowly lower back down.

Duration: 2-3 sets of 12-15 repetitions.

Benefits: Strengthens the calf muscles, improves ankle stability and balance.

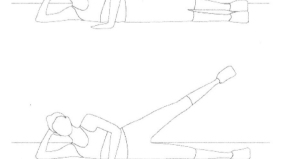

5. Wall Side Leg Lifts

How to Do It:

- Stand with your side to the wall, using the wall for balance.
- Slowly lift one leg to the side, keeping it straight then lower it back down.

Duration: 2-3 sets of 10-12 repetitions per leg.

Benefits: Works the hip abductors and glutes, enhancing hip mobility and lateral stability.

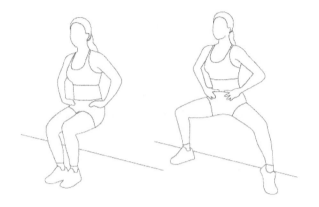

6. Wall Sit with Toe Taps

How to Do It:

- Begin in a wall sit position with your back against the wall and thighs parallel to the floor.
- Tap one foot out to the side then bring it back, followed by the other foot.

Duration: Continue alternating taps for 1-2 minutes.

Benefits: Increases the intensity of the traditional wall sit by adding movement, improving endurance in the quadriceps and challenging the hip flexors.

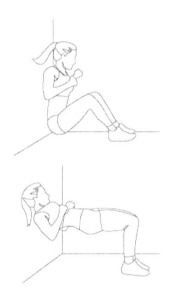

Glutes Strengthening Exercises

1. Wall Hip Thrust

How to Do It:

- Sit on the ground with your upper back against the wall, with knees bent and feet flat on the floor about hip-width apart.
- Push through your heels to lift your hips towards the ceiling, squeezing your glutes at the top.
- Lower your hips back down and repeat.

Duration: 3 sets of 12-15 repetitions.

Benefits: Targets the glutes and hamstrings, promoting hip mobility and strength.

2. Single-Leg Wall Sit

How to Do It:

- Begin in a standard wall sit position.

- Extend one leg out in front of you, holding it straight.

- Maintain the position for 20-30 seconds, then switch legs.

Duration: 2-3 sets per leg.

Benefits: Strengthens the glutes and quadriceps while challenging balance and stability.

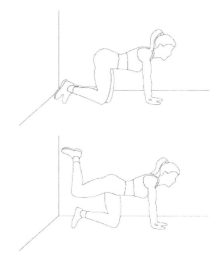

3. Wall Donkey Kicks

How to Do It:

- Start on all fours, with your feet against the wall.

- Push one heel back against the wall, driving your foot up as if trying to push the wall away.

- Return to the starting position and repeat before switching legs.

Duration: 3 sets of 10-12 repetitions per leg.

Benefits: Focuses on the glutes and helps improve lower back strength.

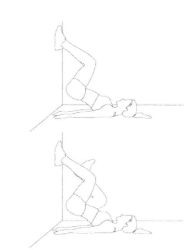

4. Wall Bridge March

How to Do It:

- Lie on your back with your feet flat against the wall and knees bent.

- Lift into a bridge position then alternate lifting each knee towards your chest in a marching motion.

Duration: 2-3 sets of 8-10 marches per leg.

Benefits: Engages the glutes and core, enhancing stability and coordination.

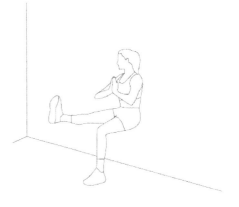

5. Diagonal Wall Squat

How to Do It:

- Stand with your back to the wall, feet wider than hip-width apart and toes turned out.

- Slide down into a squat while reaching one hand down towards the opposite foot.

- Stand back up and alternate sides.

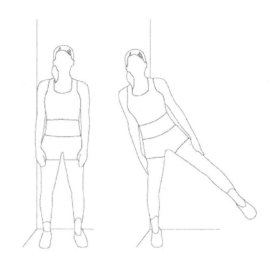

Duration: 3 sets of 10-12 repetitions.

Benefits: This exercise targets the glutes, inner thighs and obliques, improving flexibility and functional strength.

6. Wall Lateral Leg Lifts

How to Do It:

- Stand side-on to the wall, using it for balance.

- Lift the leg closest to the wall sideways while keeping your body straight then lower it back down.

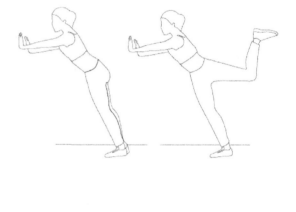

Duration: 3 sets of 12-15 repetitions per side.

Benefits: Strengthens the hip abductors and glutes, crucial for lateral movements and stability.

7. Wall Reverse Leg Lifts

How to Do It:

- Stand facing the wall, hands on the wall for support.

- Lift one leg straight behind you, keeping your hips square to the wall.

- Pause at the top then lower the leg and switch sides.

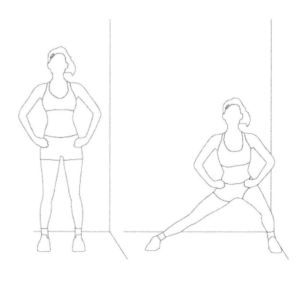

Duration: 3 sets of 10-12 repetitions per leg.

Benefits: Targets the glutes and lower back, improving posterior chain strength and posture.

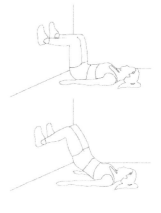

Intermediate and Advanced Lower Body Workouts

1. Wall Pistol Squats

How to Do It:

- Stand with your back against the wall, then extend one leg straight in front of you.

- Slide down the wall into a single-leg squat on the supporting leg, keeping the extended leg off the ground.

- Push through the heel to rise back up to the starting position.

Duration: 2-3 sets of 6-8 repetitions per leg.

Benefits: Develops strength and balance in the quadriceps, glutes and calves, while challenging core stability.

2. Elevated Wall Glute Bridge

How to Do It:

- Lie on your back with your feet elevated on the wall, the legs forming a 90-degree angle at the knees.

- Drive through your heels, lifting your hips off the ground while squeezing your glutes at the top.

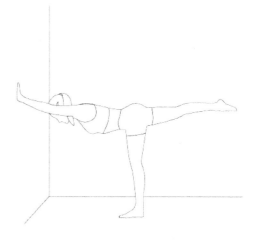

- Lower back down slowly and repeat.

Duration: 3 sets of 12-15 repetitions.

Benefits: Targets the glutes and hamstrings more intensely due to the elevated position, enhancing hip mobility and strength.

3. Wall Supported Warrior III

How to Do It:

- Stand a few feet away from the wall facing away, hinge forward at the hips and extend one leg behind you, touching the wall with your hands for balance.

- Adjust your body until it forms a T-shape, with your arms, torso and raised leg approximately parallel to the floor.

- Hold the position, then slowly return to standing and switch legs.

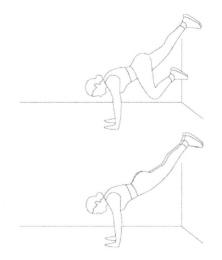

Duration: Hold for 15-20 seconds per leg for 2-3 sets.

Benefits: Improves balance and stability, strengthens the lower back, glutes and hamstrings.

4. Wall Lateral Slide Squats

How to Do It:

- Stand with your side against the wall, slide down into a squat.

- Maintain the squat position and walk sideways along the wall, taking small steps to keep the squat depth consistent.

- Move 5 steps in one direction then 5 steps back to the starting position.

Duration: 2-3 sets of 10 steps in each direction.

Benefits: Strengthens the quads, glutes and adductors, while the lateral movement adds an extra challenge to the core.

5. Inverted Wall Mountain Climbers

How to Do It:

- Place your hands on the floor in a plank position with your feet against the wall.

- Walk your feet up the wall until your body forms a 45-degree angle with the floor.

- Alternately drive each knee towards your chest in a climbing motion.

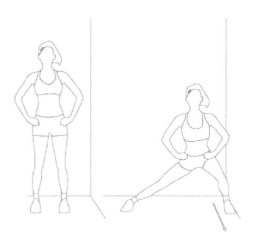

Duration: 3 sets of 15-20 repetitions per leg.

Benefits: This full-body exercise improves cardiovascular fitness, core stability and leg strength.

6. Wall Split Squat Jumps

How to Do It:

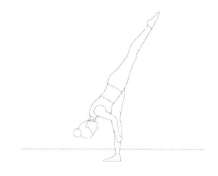

- Begin in a split squat position with your back foot elevated against the wall.

- Lower into a split squat then explosively jump up, switching legs in the air.

- Land with the opposite leg in front and the back foot against the wall and immediately lower into another split squat.

Duration: 2-3 sets of 8-10 repetitions per leg.

Benefits: Enhances power and agility in the lower body, improves cardiovascular endurance and strengthens the glutes and thighs.

Tips for Maximizing Results

It's important to schedule rest days as diligently as workout days. Muscles require at least 48 hours of recovery between strength sessions to repair micro tears from exertion. Active recovery activities like walking or gentle stretching promote circulation on rest days. Proper nutrition also helps with recovery, listen to your body and respect pain signals to prevent overtraining or acute injuries. Modify or reduce exercises that aggravate the joints, learn to build strength gradually in problem areas until you are ready to progress. Patience is key, especially when injuries or chronic conditions exist.

Record workouts to track your progress over time; logging reps, weights, sets and weekly frequency clarifies patterns and makes things easier. If plateauing, adjust variables like increasing reps first before weight. Shuffle your exercises regularly to keep challenging your muscles in fresh ways and don't forget to review your notes to stay motivated and track your progress!

Supplement Wall Pilates with complimentary activities like yoga, swimming or walking to reinforce mobility, stability and cardio endurance for cross-training benefits. Lifestyle activities like gardening, playing with kids or carrying groceries also bolster strength. It's important to note that using proper equipment also ensures safety and effectiveness when training and needs to be highlighted. Resistance bands and balls need to be inspected routinely for wear and tear and invest in thicker exercise mats to cushion knees and spine for floorwork. Wearing appropriate footwear is also necessary to maintain traction with the wall and flooring to have better exercise sessions.

Keep form cues and mental reminders visible in your workout area to anchor them in your mind. Post photos, diagrams, motivational quotes or technique tips on the wall for quick reference during your sessions. As you progress, consider adding equipment like wall ropes, ab wheels or hurdles for more advanced exercises. By creating an inspiring and functional workout space, you'll stay focused and motivated to reach your fitness goals. Nutrition cannot be overlooked for optimal strength gains, recovery and body composition. Protein repairs muscles post-workout while fruits and vegetables deliver antioxidants. It's vital to remember to hydrate well before, during and after exercise. Watching and keeping track of nutrient intake with reduced alcohol consumption will provide maximum benefits.

Above all, maintain a growth mindset. Progress through daily practice tends to be gradual rather than instantaneous. It is not something that can happen overnight, It's the accumulation of small gains over time that leads to achieving milestones you once thought were impossible. Setbacks are a natural part of the journey, learn to embrace them and strive to keep a positive mindset in the process, this will help you keep moving forward. With patience and perseverance, you'll eventually reach your goals.

The power lies within you to accomplish incredible transformation through Wall Pilates. Follow these tips to stay the course and commit fully to the process without fixating on the outcome. Consistency and self- compassion are key, you are ready to succeed.

CHAPTER 5

FLEXIBILITY AND BALANCE

Exercises to Enhance Flexibility

1. Wall Hamstring Stretch

How to Do It:

- Lie on your back close to a wall and raise one leg against the wall while keeping the other flat on the ground.

- Try to straighten the leg against the wall as much as possible to feel a stretch in the hamstring.

- Hold the position and switch legs.

Duration: Hold for 30 seconds per leg, repeat 2-3 times.

Benefits: Targets the hamstrings, enhancing flexibility and reducing tightness.

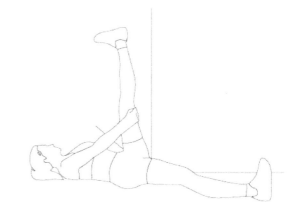

2. Wall Supported Chest Opener

How to Do It:

- Stand facing away from the wall, a few steps out. Reach back with both hands and place them flat against the wall at shoulder height.

- Slowly lean forward and lower your chest towards the ground to deepen the stretch across your chest and shoulders.

Duration: Hold for 20-30 seconds, repeat 2-3 times.

Benefits: Opens up the chest and shoulders, improving posture and respiratory function.

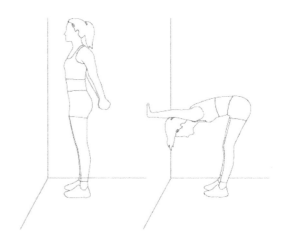

3. Vertical Wall Splits

How to Do It:

- Face the wall and place your hands on the ground for balance.
- Gradually walk your feet up the wall into a split position, going as far as your flexibility allows.

Duration: Hold for 20-30 seconds, repeat 2-3 times.

Benefits: Increases flexibility in the hamstrings and hip flexors, promotes better circulation in the lower limbs.

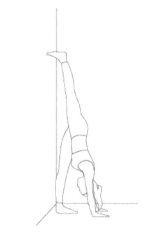

4. Wall Supported Warrior Pose

How to Do It:

- Stand a couple of feet away from a wall. Extend one foot back and place it flat against the wall.
- Bend the front knee to enter into a warrior pose, ensuring the knee does not extend past the toes.
- Raise your arms above your head or place them on your hips.

Duration: Hold for 20-30 seconds per side, repeat 2-3 times.

Benefits: Stretches the hip flexors, improves balance and stability, and strengthens lower body muscles.

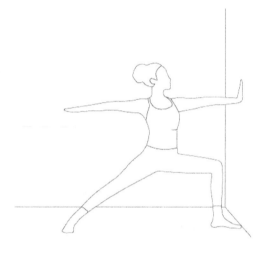

5. Wall Angel

How to Do It:

- Press your arms against the wall with elbows bent, like the hands of a clock at 9:15.
- Slowly slide your arms up to form a "Y" and then bring them down, maintaining contact with the wall.

Duration: Repeat for 10-12 repetitions, 2-3 sets.

Benefits: Improves shoulder mobility and stretches the upper back, helps correct posture issues.

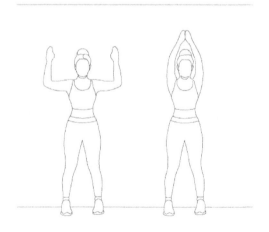

6. Wall-Assisted Downward Dog

How to Do It:

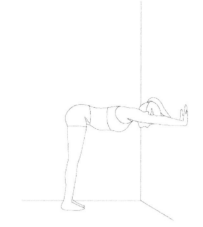

- Place your hands on the wall at waist height.

- Step back until your body forms an inverted V shape, with your head between your arms.

- Push your chest towards the floor to deepen the stretch.

Duration: Hold for 20-30 seconds, repeat 2-3 times.

Benefits: Stretches the spine, shoulders and hamstrings; increases overall body flexibility and relieves back tension.

Balance Improvement Techniques

Balance requires integration of multiple body systems. This involves vestibular, visual, proprioception, cardiovascular and muscular. Pilates builds strength, proprioception and coordination to enhance stability and control. Maintaining equilibrium improves daily function and reduces falls, especially as people grow older. These techniques develop balance safely.

Start by assessing your current capabilities. Measure the time you can stand on one leg with your eyes open, then repeat the test with your eyes closed to establish a baseline. Check both your right and left sides, any asymmetry suggests areas that need specific attention. Trying simple moves like the tandem stance or toe raises can help pinpoint problem areas for further focus and improvement. Start exercises near a wall for support as needed. Lightly touching a surface while lifting a foot can help build confidence before attempting to do hands-free balancing. Standing side-kicks, using the wall for support, target stabilizing leg muscles while providing stability. As your balance improves, gradually decrease the contact with the wall to challenge yourself even further.

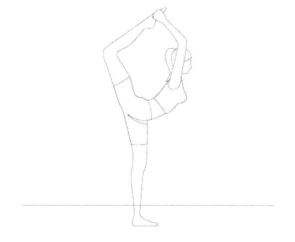

Utilize small, controlled motions to keep yourself centered over your base of support. Incorporating mini-squats helps maintain smooth and aligned movements. Lateral steps and crossover steps can be added subsequently once stability has been established. Only increase the range of motion within your ability to maintain control and proper form. Try to incorporate dynamic upper body movements like arm raises or circles, integrating limbs helps improves motor coordination. Using rubber resistance bands held in both hands introduces multidirectional variable challenges, helping to train reactions and improve overall strength.

Advance to unstable surfaces such as foam pads, cushions or balance boards when you are ready. These surfaces engage more leg muscles to maintain stability as they compress. Always have an emergency contact nearby to help until you feel confident with your balance. You can practice balancing during daily activities, that is, in real life situations. For example, you can do this by standing on one foot while washing the dishes or brushing your teeth, walking heel to toe along a line on the ground or getting up slowly from chairs without using any of your hands. You can also do this by closing your eyes once you are in a comfortable and steady position to eliminate vision and then shift your weight subtly between your feet, engaging the core muscles to stay upright. Cues like sound, touch and verbal instruction can guide movement in the absence of sight.

The mind-body connection is crucial for balance. Direct your focus inward, paying attention to your body position, muscle activation and intention. Cultivating meditative qualities fosters equilibrium between tension and relaxation, allowing for graceful movement. Patience is vital in balance training to prevent frustration or injury. It is normal to expect gradual gains through daily practice. Small successes build physical capability, mental and emotional confidence over time. Simply standing tall and aligned fosters poise. Consistency ultimately results in fluidity of motion, precision and embodiment. The mind guides movement harmoniously between stillness and motion. With practice, Pilates balance training develops poise, presence and postural control.

Integrating Flexibility and Balance into Everyday Activities

Life often feels busy, leaving fitness relegated to structured workouts. Yet simple ways exist to incorporate Pilates principles into daily routines. Subtle shifts build mobility, stability and mind-body awareness throughout the day. Morning routines prime the body and mind for the upcoming day. Wake up a few minutes early to flow through sun salutations, engaging every muscle group. Balance on one foot while brushing teeth, stretch fingertips overhead and lengthening the sides of the waist by stretching. Move with intention. Commuting provides opportunities for mobility exercises. You can perform neck rolls at stoplights to reduce tension, alternate ankle circles while on public transportation. Stretching the hips, hamstrings and calves keeps your muscles supple after sitting especially if you have been sitting for quite some time. Taking occasional deep breaths is also very necessary.

The workplace generally requires significant stationary sitting. Every 30-60 minutes, stand up and open your hips to reverse hip flexor tightness. Incorporate shoulder rolls and wrist circles to feel freer and more refreshed. Having walking meetings helps build more body movement and creates a space for clearer thinking. Errands and household chores are also pretty great for training functional fitness. When unloading groceries or a laundry basket, make sure to squat properly, this helps to activate your glutes and thighs. Vacuuming or mopping can strengthen your upper back muscles. Gardening allows for a full range of motion and engagement of various muscle groups. Don't forget about carrying children, this is a great way to connect with them while also providing a workout for your arms and core.

Of course, scheduling dedicated flexibility sessions provide maximum benefits. Sustain stretches for 30 to 90 seconds, focusing on tight areas such as the hip flexors, hamstrings and chest. Utilize props like straps or foam rollers as needed to enhance your stretches. Feel the tension release as you hold each stretch.

Preparing for dinner also engages core strength and balance. You can stand on one leg while chopping vegetables, alternating sides while doing so. Wipe countertops without arching the low back and do calf raises while washing the dishes to energize the lower body after a long day. In the evening, unwind tight muscles from stress or prolonged postures. Restorative yoga poses, gentle rolling and light stretching can help restore length to your muscles. When watching television, support your neck and lower back to maintain good posture. Remember to stay hydrated throughout the day to support your body's recovery and overall well-being.

Before heading to bed, standing balance poses can help to keep a calm mind. Sway gently side to side, anchoring through the arches of the feet. Turn off screens well before bedtime to help facilitate better sleep. Allow yourself to let go of the events of the day, creating a peaceful and relaxed environment conducive to restful sleep. With planning, Pilates enhances every part of daily life, it is not a just form of exercise. Integrating movement with purposeful pauses shapes your fitness journey over time. Consistency in practice develops awareness, mobility and a deeper connection with your body. Embrace the essence of Pilates in your daily life, embodying its principles fully.

Challenges to Test Your Progress

Pilates cultivates physical and mental capabilities over time through consistent practice. Testing your progress periodically provides motivation while highlighting areas needing more focus and attention. These challenges improve stamina, control, mobility and confidence. With patience and commitment, you will surprise yourself at how your abilities evolve over time. Standing balance poses held for a specific amount of time provide an objective measurement of progress. Start with shorter durations, such as 30 seconds and gradually increase to a minute then 5 minutes and eventually 10 minutes over the course of several months. Notice how stillness deepens and wavering subsides with practice.

Aim to effortlessly stand tall on one leg with stability and grace as you progress. Planks and variations like side planks help build core endurance. Each week, record the duration for which you can maintain proper form while breathing fully during standing balance poses. Strong core muscles help prevent compensations, allowing for longer holds. Experiment with varying hand and foot positions to challenge yourself further. As you become more proficient, consider transitioning between standing and balancing on your elbows for additional progression. A full range of motion reveals increased flexibility over time. Measure progress by stretching hamstrings, chest, shoulders and hips using pictures taken over time or simply by using your hands. Reaching farther to touch your toes or clasping your hands behind your back demonstrates opening. Move to your edge, not past it.

Wall squat holds are effective for incrementally strengthening your legs. Begin by lowering into the squat position until your thighs are parallel to the ground, then time how long you can maintain proper form. Gradually increase the duration of the holds by 5-10 seconds and add more repetitions as you progress. Proper activation of the glutes helps reduce strain on the knees and lower back during the exercise. Moving plank walks build coordination with integrating the limbs. Start by counting how many steps you can take while maintaining stability and proper alignment. Only increase the distance and speed of your steps when you can do so while still maintaining perfect technique.

 This gradual approach ensures that you prioritize technique over speed or distance, leading to safer and more effective progress. Sharpen the mind-body connection through fluid transitions. The Hundred is great for boosting cardio capacity and testing endurance. Begin by keeping your legs suspended and pulsing your arms with controlled breaths for 100 counts initially. This exercise challenges both your cardiovascular system and your muscular endurance, making it an energizing addition to any workout routine. Add repetitions over weeks and months for more definition, sculpted abs and stamina. Maintain lifting your legs without putting tension on your neck.

Balance squat holds combine stability challenges. From a standing position, get lower into a squat position with your arms extended. Hold for 10 breaths then return upright with control. Gradually increase squat depth and hold duration to master the exercise, while maintaining a neutral spine. Recording and reviewing periodic progress provides perspective on subtle shifts over time. Small measurable gains reinforce commitment. Prioritize integrity by utilizing the full range of motion in your movements. Remember, numbers should serve as guides, not as goals in and of themselves. Overall poise emerges from regular practice.

Notice your increased ability to move with precision and ease after each practice. Observe improved posture and a grounded presence, confidence arises from the embodiment cultivated through Wall Pilates over time. Know that plateaus are natural, you can adjust the intensity or intervals to stimulate further adaptation. Deepen mind-body awareness to bypass limitations. Focus on the journey, not just the destination, progress manifests through consistent practice. Trust in your growing strength, mobility and balance and regularly test your evolution to stay motivated. With dedication, the challenges that once seemed impossible will be conquered with patience and compassion. Believe in your potential. You are strong.

CHAPTER 6

FULL BODY WORKOUTS

A comprehensive Wall Pilates routine strengthens all major muscle groups for balanced fitness. Thoughtful programming provides variation, progression and recovery to maximize benefits safely. These guidelines help to craft an effective full body flow.

Sample Beginner Full Body Workouts

1. Wall Push-Ups

How to Do It:

- Stand facing the wall at arm's length.

- Place your hands on the wall slightly wider than shoulder-width apart.

- Bend your elbows to lower your chest towards the wall, then push back to the starting position.

Duration: 2-3 sets of 10-12 repetitions.

Benefits: Strengthens the chest, shoulders and triceps. Easier on the wrists and shoulders than floor push-ups.

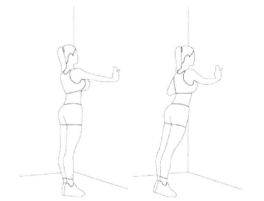

2. Wall Squats

How to Do It:

- Stand with your back against the wall, feet shoulder-width apart, about two feet from the wall.

- Slide down the wall until your knees are at 90 degrees.

- Hold the position then slide back up. Ensure your back remains flat against the wall throughout.

Duration: 2-3 sets of 10-15 repetitions.

Benefits: Targets the quadriceps, hamstrings and glutes while helping to improve lower body strength and endurance.

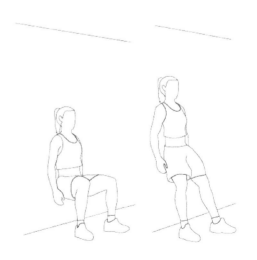

3. Wall Pelvic Tilts

How to Do It:

- Stand with your back against the wall, feet shoulder-width apart.

- Press the small of your back into the wall by tilting your pelvis forward.

- Hold for a few seconds then return to the starting position.

Duration: 2-3 sets of 12-15 repetitions.

Benefits: Strengthens the abdominal muscles and lower back, improves posture and enhances core stability.

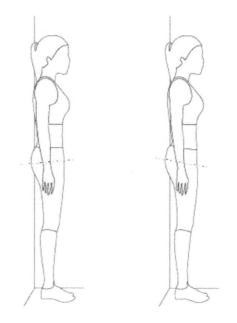

4. Standing Wall Leg Lifts

How to Do It:

- Stand side-on to the wall with your hand for support.

- Slowly lift the leg closest to the wall up to the side, keeping it straight.

- Hold briefly at the top then lower back down without touching the floor.

Duration: 2-3 sets of 10-12 repetitions per leg.

Benefits: Improves balance and coordination, strengthens the hip abductors and core muscles.

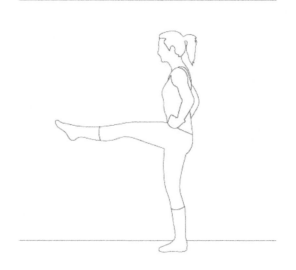

5. Wall Calf Raises

How to Do It:

- Face the wall and stand arm's length away. Place hands on the wall for balance.

- Lift your heels off the ground, rising onto your toes.

- Hold briefly then slowly lower your heels back to the floor.

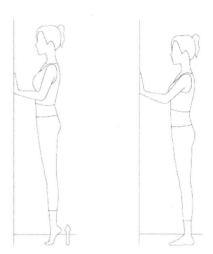

Duration: 2-3 sets of 15-20 repetitions.

Benefits: Strengthens the calf muscles, improves ankle stability and balance.

6. Wall Plank

How to Do It:

- Face the wall and stand a few feet away from it.

- Lean forward and place your forearms on the wall, keeping elbows below shoulders.

- Step back until your body forms a straight line from head to heels.

Duration: Hold for 20-30 seconds, 2-3 sets.

Benefits: Engages the entire core, including the abdominals and lower back, enhancing core strength and stability.

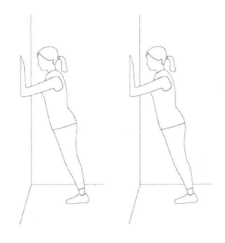
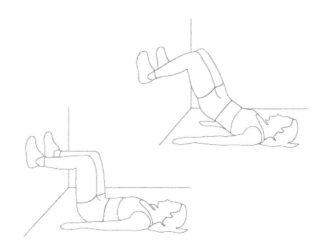

Sample Intermediate Full Body Workouts

1. Wall Bridge

How to Do It:

- Lie on your back with your feet flat against the wall, knees bent at a 90-degree angle.
- Lift your hips to create a straight line from your shoulders to your knees.
- Hold the position then slowly lower your hips back to the floor.

Duration: 3 sets of 10-15 repetitions.

Benefits: Strengthens the glutes, hamstrings and lower back, while engaging the core.

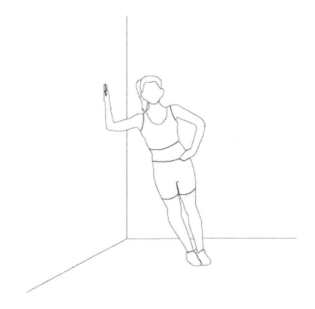

2. Side Wall Plank

How to Do It:

- Start by lying on one side with your feet against the wall and your elbow directly under your shoulder.

- Lift your hips off the ground, forming a straight line from head to feet and press your feet against the wall for stability.

- Hold the position, then switch sides.

Duration: Hold for 30-45 seconds per side, 2-3 sets.

Benefits: Strengthens the obliques, shoulders and core while improving balance.

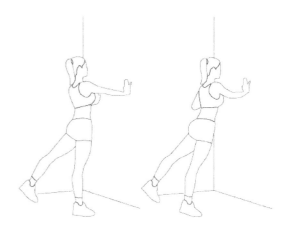

3. Wall Push-Up with Leg Lift

How to Do It:

- Stand facing the wall at arm's length, place your hands on the wall at shoulder height.

- As you perform a push-up against the wall, lift one leg off the ground.

- Alternate the lifted leg with each repetition.

Duration: 2-3 sets of 10-12 repetitions.

Benefits: Enhances coordination and balance, strengthens the chest, triceps and core, and also increases lower body stability.

4. Wall Mountain Climbers

How to Do It:

- Place your hands on the floor about 2 feet from the wall.

- Extend your legs and place your toes against the wall, similar to a plank position.

- Alternately drive each knee towards your chest rapidly, as if climbing.

Duration: 3 sets of 30 seconds to 1 minute.

Benefits: Provides a cardiovascular workout, strengthens the core and enhances agility and coordination.

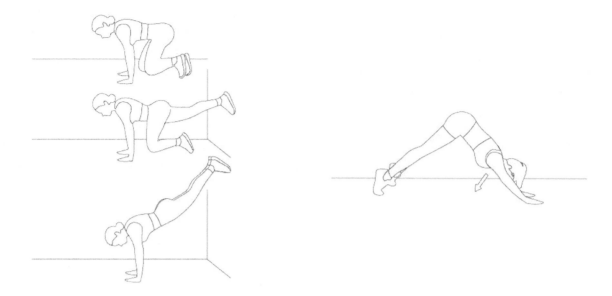

5. Inverted Wall V-Press

How to Do It:

- Start in a handstand position with your feet against the wall.
- Bend your elbows to lower your head towards the ground then press back up.
- Ensure your core is engaged to maintain balance.

Duration: 2-3 sets of 6-8 repetitions.

Benefits: Builds upper body strength, particularly in the shoulders and arms, and improves balance and core stability.

6. Wall-Assisted Pistol Squats

How to Do It:

- Stand with your back to the wall and walk your feet out slightly.
- Extend one leg in front of you and lower yourself into a squat on the supporting leg, sliding down the wall for support.
- Push back up and repeat then switch legs.

Duration: 2-3 sets of 8-10 repetitions per leg.

Benefits: Targets the quadriceps, glutes and calves, improves balance and unilateral (single-leg) strength.

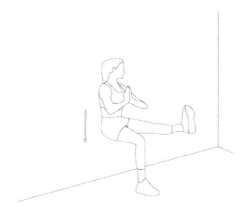 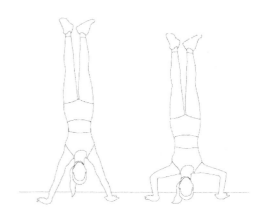

Sample Advanced Full Body Workouts

1. Wall-Assisted Handstand Push-Ups

How to Do It:

- Begin in a handstand position with your back against the wall.

- Lower your body by bending your elbows until your head nearly touches the floor.

- Push back up to the starting position.

Duration: 2-3 sets of 5-8 repetitions.

Benefits: Strengthens shoulders, arms and core, while improving balance and upper body endurance.

2. One-Legged Wall Squat

How to Do It:

- Lift one foot off the ground, extending it forward.

- Lower into a squat on the supporting leg, sliding down the wall.

- Return to the starting position and switch legs.

Duration: 2-3 sets of 8-10 repetitions per leg.

Benefits: Enhances lower body strength and balance, particularly in the quadriceps, hamstrings and glutes.

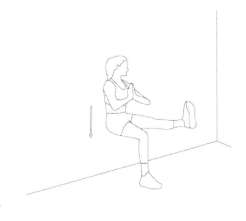
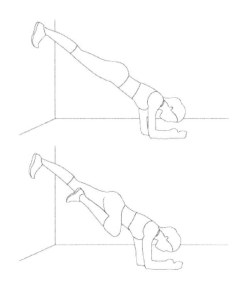

3. Wall Plank with Leg Thread

How to Do It:

- Start in a forearm plank with your feet against the wall.
- Rotate your hips and thread one leg under your body and through to the opposite side, keeping it off the ground.
- Return to the starting position and repeat with the other leg.

Duration: 2-3 sets of 10-12 repetitions per side.

Benefits: Increases core strength and stability, enhances rotational mobility and engages the entire body.

4. Wall Reverse Plank

How to Do It:

- Sit on the ground with your back towards the wall and your legs extended forward.
- Place your hands on the ground behind you and lift your body to form a straight line from head to heels, with heels pressing against the wall.
- Hold the position, maintaining a rigid body line.

Duration: Hold for 30-45 seconds, 2-3 sets.

Benefits: Strengthens the posterior chain including the lower back, glutes and hamstrings, and improves posture.

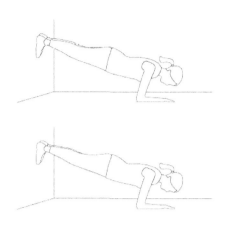

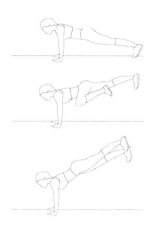

5. Wall Lateral Climbs

How to Do It:

- Begin in a push-up position with your side facing the wall and feet placed against the base of the wall.

- Move laterally along the wall using your hands and feet, maintaining a plank position.

- Move for a set distance or number of steps then return in the opposite direction.

Duration: 2-3 sets of 5-10 lateral movements each direction.

Benefits: Builds core stability, upper body strength and coordination.

6. Vertical Wall Run

How to Do It:

- Stand facing the wall at a distance where you can place your hands on the wall at waist height.

- Quickly alternate bringing your knees up towards the wall as if running vertically.

Duration: 3 sets of 20-30 seconds.

Benefits: Improves cardiovascular fitness, enhances leg strength and speed, and builds core stability.

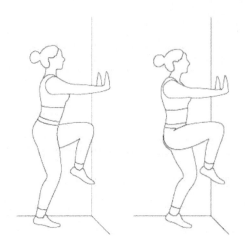

CHAPTER 7

SPECIAL PILATES ROUTINES FOR SPECIFIC NEEDS

Pilates for Back Pain Relief

1. Wall Pelvic Tilt

How to Do It:

- Stand with your back against the wall, feet shoulder-width apart and slightly away from the wall.

- Flatten your lower back against the wall by gently tilting your pelvis.

- Hold for a few seconds then return to the starting position.

Duration: 3 sets of 10 repetitions.

Benefits: Helps realign the pelvis and strengthen the lower abdominal muscles, reducing lower back strain.

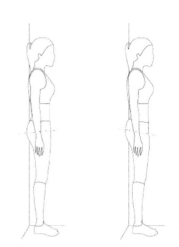

2. Wall Supported Cat-Cow

How to Do It:

- Stand a few feet away from the wall, leaning forward to place your hands on the wall at shoulder height.

- As you inhale, arch your back downward, lifting your head and tailbone towards the ceiling (Cow position).

- As you exhale, round your spine towards the wall, dropping your head and tailbone (Cat position).

Duration: 3 sets of 8-10 repetitions.

Benefits: Increases spinal flexibility and eases tension in the torso, promoting mobility and relief in the back.

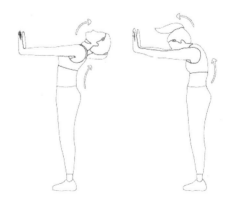

3. Wall Standing Leg Extension

How to Do It:

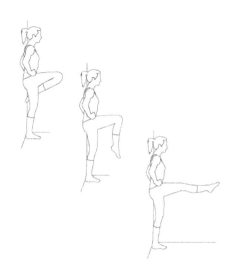

- Stand with your back to the wall, feet hip-width apart.

- Press one foot into the wall at hip height to stabilize then gently lift the opposite knee towards your chest.

- Slowly extend the lifted leg forward, keeping your back flat against the wall.

- Return to the bent knee position and switch legs.

Duration: 2 sets of 8-10 repetitions per leg.

Benefits: Strengthens the core and lower back while improving leg flexibility and balance.

4. Wall Supported Bridge

How to Do It:

- Lie on your back with your arms at your sides, knees bent and feet flat against the wall.

- Lift your hips towards the ceiling, pressing your feet into the wall and arms into the ground for support.

- Hold the position for a few seconds then slowly lower your hips back to the floor.

Duration: 3 sets of 10-12 repetitions.

Benefits: Strengthens the glutes and lower back, which are crucial for supporting the spine.

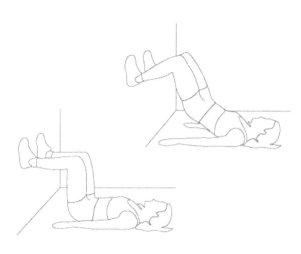

5. Wall Slide Squats

How to Do It:

- Stand with your back against the wall, feet shoulder-width apart.

- Slide down into a squat position until your knees are bent at a 90-degree angle.

- Hold the squat for a few seconds then slide back up.

Duration: 3 sets of 10 repetitions.

Benefits: Strengthens the thighs and buttocks while reducing stress on the lower back.

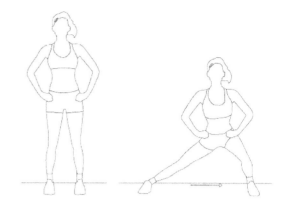

6. Wall Clock Stretch

How to Do It:

- Stand facing the wall, extend your right arm and place your hand on the wall at shoulder height.

- Slowly move your hand in a clock-like motion from 12 to 3 and back, feeling the stretch in your shoulder and side of your back.

- Repeat on the left side.

Duration: 2 sets of 5 repetitions per arm.

Benefits: Enhances shoulder flexibility and releases tension in the upper and middle back.

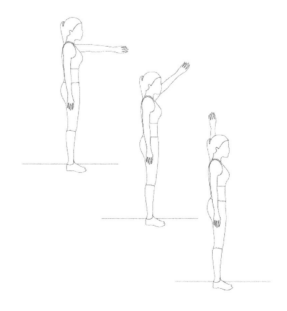

Post-pregnancy Pilates Workouts

1. Wall-Assisted Pelvic Tilt

How to Do It:

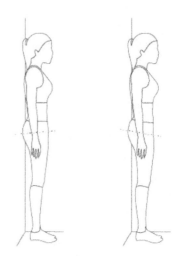

- Stand with your back against the wall, feet hip-width apart.

- Keep your spine neutral and gently press your lower back into the wall by tilting your pelvis.

- Hold for a few seconds then release gently.

Duration: 3 sets of 10 repetitions.

Benefits: Helps to strengthen the pelvic floor and lower abdominal muscles, aids in realigning and stabilizing the pelvis post-pregnancy.

2. Wall Supported Squat

How to Do It:

- Stand with your back against the wall, feet shoulder-width apart and a step away from the wall.

- Lower into a squat while sliding down the wall, ensuring your knees do not extend past your toes.

- Hold the squat position briefly then slide back up.

Duration: 2-3 sets of 8-10 repetitions.

Benefits: Strengthens quads, hamstrings, glutes and core, while being gentle on the joints.

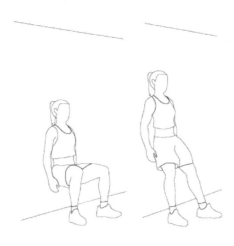

3. Wall Push-ups

How to Do It:

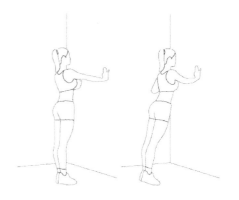

- Stand at arm's length away from the wall with feet together.

- Place your hands on the wall at shoulder height and width.

- Bend your elbows to bring your chest towards the wall, then push back to the starting position.

Duration: 2-3 sets of 10-12 repetitions.

Benefits: Builds upper body strength and tones arms without straining the back, important for handling baby care tasks.

4. Wall Leg Slide

How to Do It:

- Lie on your side near the wall, with your back against the wall.

- Keep your bottom leg bent for stability and your top leg straight.

- Slide the top leg up the wall while keeping it straight then slide it back down.

Duration: 2 sets of 8-10 repetitions on each side.

Benefits: Helps in strengthening the inner and outer thighs, improves hip mobility, and stabilizes pelvic muscles.

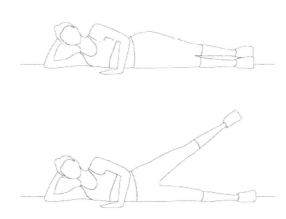

5. Wall-Assisted Standing Knee Lift

How to Do It:

- Stand facing the wall with your hands on the wall for balance.

- Slowly lift one knee towards the chest without bending the supporting leg or shifting hips.

- Hold briefly, then lower the knee and switch sides.

Duration: 2-3 sets of 8-10 repetitions per leg.

Benefits: Enhances core stability and balance, strengthens lower abdominals and pelvic floor muscles.

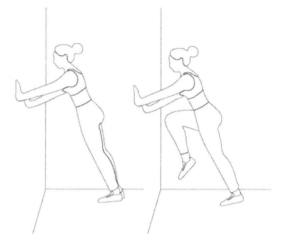

6. Wall Supported Back Stretch

How to Do It:

- Stand facing away from the wall, a few feet away and lean back until your hands reach the wall, keeping them at hip level.

- Bend your knees slightly and push your hips forward, arching your back gently against the wall.

Duration: Hold for 20-30 seconds, repeat 2-3 times.

Benefits: Stretches and relaxes the lower back muscles, helping to alleviate postural stress from nursing and carrying the baby.

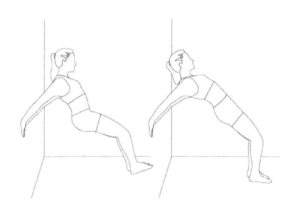

Pilates for Aging Women

1. Wall Supported Roll Down

How to Do It:

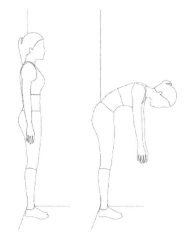

- Stand with your back against the wall, feet hip-width apart and slightly away from the wall.

- Slowly roll down the wall by tucking your chin to your chest and peeling your spine off the wall, one vertebra at a time, until you reach a comfortable bent-over position.

- Slowly roll back up to the starting position.

Duration: 2-3 sets of 6-8 repetitions.

Benefits: Enhances spinal mobility and gently stretches the back muscles, promoting better posture and flexibility.

2. Wall Angel

How to Do It:

- Stand with your back against the wall, feet slightly forward with knees slightly bent.

- Press your arms against the wall with elbows bent and slide them up and down, mimicking a snow angel motion.

Duration: 2-3 sets of 8-10 repetitions.

Benefits: Improves shoulder mobility and strengthens the upper back and scapular muscles, which are crucial for everyday activities.

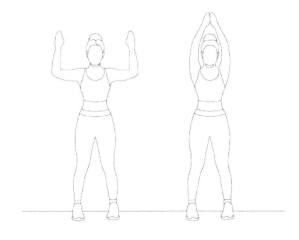

3. Wall Supported Side Leg Lift

How to Do It:

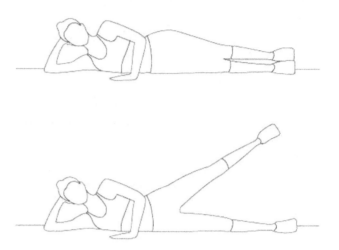

- Stand side-on to the wall, placing your hand on the wall for support.

- Keep your standing leg slightly bent for stability and lift the other leg sideways, keeping it straight.

- Hold briefly at the top then lower the leg with control.

Duration: 2 sets of 8-10 repetitions per leg.

Benefits: Strengthens the hips and stabilizes the pelvic muscles, which help in maintaining balance and preventing falls.

4. Wall Assisted Calf Raises

How to Do It:

- Stand facing the wall with hands on the wall for balance.

- Lift your heels off the ground, rising onto your toes.

- Hold briefly, then lower back down.

Duration: 3 sets of 10-12 repetitions.

Benefits: Strengthens the calf muscles and improves ankle stability, essential for walking and climbing stairs.

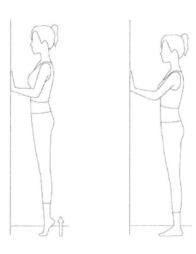

5. Wall Plank

How to Do It:

- Stand facing the wall, place your hands on the wall at shoulder height.

- Walk your feet back until your body forms a straight line from head to heels, leaning into the wall.

Duration: Hold for 20-30 seconds, repeat 2-3 times.

Benefits: Strengthens the core and shoulders, improves overall body stability and builds endurance in a safe manner.

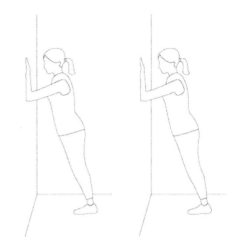

Wall Supported Chair Pose

How to Do It:

- Stand with your back against the wall.

- Slide down into a seated position, as if sitting in a chair, with knees bent at a 90-degree angle.

- Try to hold this position, keeping the thighs parallel to the floor.

Duration: Hold for 20-30 seconds, repeat 2-3 times.

Benefits: Strengthens the thighs, buttocks and core, enhancing lower body strength and improving balance.

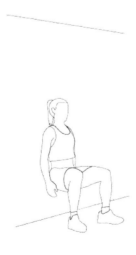

Pilates as Stress Relief

1. Wall Slide Breathing

How to Do It:

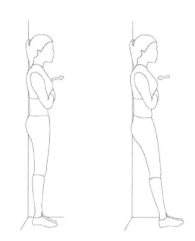

- Stand with your back flat against the wall, feet slightly away from the wall.

- Place your hands on your lower ribcage.

- Inhale deeply, expanding your ribs laterally, while sliding your hands up toward your chest.

- Exhale slowly, sliding your hands back down to the starting position.

Duration: 2-3 minutes of continuous, deep breathing.

Benefits: Helps improve lung capacity and diaphragmatic breathing, reduces physical and mental tension.

2. Wall Supported Tree Pose

How to Do It:

- Stand next to the wall with your side facing the wall for balance.

- Shift your weight onto one leg and place the sole of your other foot on your inner thigh or calf (avoid the knee).

- Rest one hand on the wall and bring the other to a prayer position at your chest.

Duration: Hold for 30 seconds to 1 minute then switch sides.

Benefits: Enhances balance and focus, calms the mind and reduces stress.

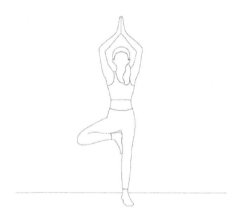

3. Wall Supported Forward Bend

How to Do It:

- Face the wall, standing about two feet away.
- Hinge at the hips to fold forward, placing your hands on the wall at hip height.
- Let your head hang loosely and relax your neck.

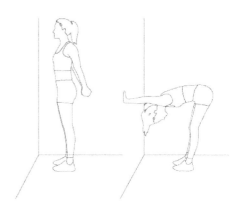

Duration: Hold for 30 seconds to 1 minute.

Benefits: Stretches the back and hamstrings, releases tension in the spine and neck, promotes relaxation.

4. Wall Butterfly Stretch

How to Do It:

- Sit on the floor with your back against the wall, knees bent and soles of the feet together.
- Let your knees fall open to the sides.
- Gently press your knees toward the ground using your elbows for an added stretch.

Duration: Hold for 1-2 minutes.

Benefits: Opens the hips and lower back, helps relieve stress and tension in the pelvic area, promotes a sense of grounding.

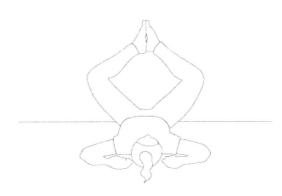

5. Wall Roll Down

How to Do It:

- Stand with your back to the wall, feet hip-width apart and about 6 inches from the wall.

- Slowly roll down the wall, vertebra by vertebra, starting from your head, allowing your neck and shoulders to fully relax.

- Hang at the bottom with your arms loose for a few breaths then slowly roll back up.

Duration: Repeat 3-5 times.

Benefits: Calms the nervous system, stretches the spine and releases tension throughout the body.

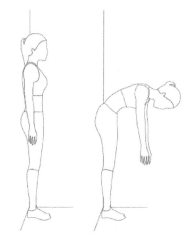

6. Wall Supported Warrior Pose

How to Do It:

- Stand in a warrior II position with one side of your body close to the wall, using the wall for balance if needed.

- Extend your arms out to the sides, with one arm touching the wall for support.

- Focus on a deep, steady breath, maintaining the position.

Duration: Hold for 30 seconds to 1 minute on each side.

Benefits: Builds focus and stamina, reduces stress, stretches and tones the legs and hips.

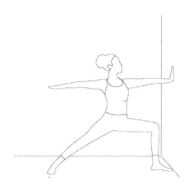

CHAPTER 8

NUTRITION AND PILATES

Basic Nutrition for Pilates Practitioners

Proper nutrition provides the foundation for Pilates training as well as a healthy, active lifestyle. Quality fuel maximizes energy, provides good recovery and achieves results. Being mindful of eating habits can support overall well-being beyond the mat. Explore other ways to nourish your body optimally, Hydration is essential. Drink enough water before, during and after each workout session. Dehydration causes fatigue, cramping and strained joints. Aim for at least 64 ounces per day, more if you are sweating heavily. Herbal tea and diluted juices also contribute to fluid goals.

Eat a rainbow of anti-inflammatory fruits and vegetables. The antioxidants, vitamins and minerals aid muscle repair while boosting immunity. Focus more on leafy greens, berries, citrus fruits and squash. Prep produce simply; fresh, roasted, juiced or blended into smoothies. Lean proteins like chicken, fish, eggs, legumes, nuts and seeds satisfy hunger while rebuilding muscles. Aim for 20-30 grams of protein within 30 minutes after training for effective recovery.

Enjoy sustainable seafood and plant proteins often. Healthy fats provide lasting energy and lubricate the joints. Incorporate essential fatty acids and vitamin E into your diet with nuts, seeds, avocado, olive oil, and fatty fish. Opt for plant oils instead of butter for cooking. Steer clear of trans and saturated fats, which can trigger inflammation. Complex carbohydrates offer sustained fuel for active bodies. Whole grains like quinoa, brown rice, oats and sprouted bread support training while providing fiber. Limit your intake of simple carbohydrates, as excess sugar can lead to energy crashes. Be mindful of when you consume carbohydrates and time your intake appropriately throughout the day.

Nourish a healthy gut micro biome with fermented foods. Yogurt, kefir, kimchi, sauerkraut and kombucha contain probiotics for digestion and immunity. Reduce inflammatory foods that may cause sensitivities like gluten, dairy and alcohol. Avoid sugary sports drinks that may cause stomach upset, refuel intelligently after training. Prepare nutrient-dense meals and snacks rather than relying on supplements alone Supplements can however, address specific individual needs under a doctor's guidance. Whole foods provide a complex array of vitamins, minerals and phytonutrients. Treat yourself in moderation.

Allow room occasionally for favorite treats without feeling any guilt. Notice how certain foods leave you feeling, aim for those that provide more of energy and satisfaction. You deserve nourishment and joy. Consistency with nutrition empowers the Pilates practice. Proper fueling and hydration amplifies its benefits. Feed yourself wholesome, delicious foods that vitalize your body. Let food be thy medicine through conscientious choices.

Breakfast Recipes

Banana and Almond Butter Toast

For: 2 people

Ingredients:

4 slices whole-grain bread

2 ripe bananas

4 tablespoons almond butter

1 teaspoon chia seeds

Preparation:

Toast the bread slices to your preference.

Spread a tablespoon of almond butter on each slice.

Slice bananas and lay them over the almond butter.

Sprinkle chia seeds on top of the bananas.

Preparation Time: 10 minutes

Benefits: Provides a good mix of protein, healthy fats and fiber. Almond butter offers vitamin E and magnesium, while bananas provide potassium, aiding in muscle recovery and energy levels.

Greek Yogurt Parfait with Mixed Berries and Granola

For: 2 people

Ingredients:

2 cups Greek yogurt

1 cup mixed berries (blueberries, strawberries, raspberries)

1 cup granola

2 tablespoons honey

Preparation:

In two glasses, layer Greek yogurt, mixed berries and granola.

Repeat the layers until the glasses are filled.

Drizzle honey over the top.

Preparation Time: 5 minutes

Benefits: High in protein and probiotics from the yogurt, which support digestive health. Berries add antioxidants and granola provides a satisfying crunch and fiber.

Spinach and Mushroom Omelette

For: 2 people

Ingredients:

6 eggs

1 cup chopped spinach

1 cup sliced mushrooms

1/2 cup shredded cheese (optional)

Salt and pepper to taste

1 tablespoon olive oil

Preparation:

Heat olive oil in a skillet over medium heat.

Sauté mushrooms until they are soft.

Add spinach and cook until wilted.

Beat eggs and pour over the vegetables in the skillet

Sprinkle cheese on top and season with salt and pepper.

Cook until the eggs are set and fold the omelette before serving.

Preparation Time: 15 minutes

Benefits: Eggs provide high-quality protein, essential for muscle repair. Spinach and mushrooms are excellent sources of vitamins and minerals, supporting overall health and energy.

Avocado and Egg Breakfast Salad

For: 2 people

Ingredients:

4 hard-boiled eggs, sliced

1 large avocado, diced

2 cups mixed salad greens

1/2 of cucumber, sliced

2 tablespoons olive oil

1 tablespoon lemon juice

Salt and pepper to taste

Preparation:

In a large bowl, combine salad greens, sliced cucumber and diced avocado.

Add sliced hard-boiled eggs.

In a small bowl, whisk together olive oil, lemon juice, salt and pepper.

Drizzle the dressing over the salad and toss gently.

Preparation Time: 10 minutes

Benefits: Loaded with healthy fats from avocado and olive oil. Eggs add protein, while greens provide fiber and micronutrients for a balanced start.

Blueberry and Walnut Oatmeal

For: 2 people

Ingredients:

1 cup rolled oats

2 cups water or milk

1 cup fresh blueberries

1/2 cup walnuts, chopped

2 tablespoons maple syrup or honey

Preparation:

In a saucepan, bring water or milk to a boil.

Add oats and reduce heat to simmer, stirring occasionally until oats are soft.

Stir in blueberries and walnuts, and cook for another 2 minutes.

Serve with a drizzle of maple syrup or honey.

Preparation Time: 10 minutes

Benefits: Oats are a great source of soluble fiber, aiding in digestion and sustained energy release. Blueberries are rich in antioxidants and walnuts provide omega-3 fatty acids, supporting brain health.

Lunch Recipes

Quinoa Chickpea Salad

For: 2 people

Ingredients:

1 cup cooked quinoa

1 cup canned chickpeas, rinsed and drained

1 small cucumber, diced

1 bell pepper, diced

1/4 cup chopped red onion

1/4 cup feta cheese, crumbled

2 tablespoons olive oil

Juice of 1 lemon

Salt and pepper to taste

Preparation:

In a large bowl, mix the cooked quinoa, chickpeas, cucumber, bell pepper and red onion.

Add the feta cheese.

In a small bowl, whisk together olive oil, lemon juice, salt and pepper.

Pour the dressing over the salad and toss to combine.

Preparation Time: 15 minutes

Benefits: This salad is rich in plant-based protein from quinoa and chickpeas, making it great for muscle repair and recovery. The variety of vegetables provides essential vitamins and antioxidants, while olive oil delivers healthy fats.

Turkey and Avocado Wrap

For: 2 people

Ingredients:

4 whole wheat tortillas

8 slices turkey breast

1 ripe avocado, sliced

1 cup mixed greens

1 tomato, sliced

1/4 cup mayonnaise or Greek yogurt

Salt and pepper to taste

Preparation:

Lay out the tortillas and spread each with mayonnaise or Greek yogurt.

Layer turkey slices, avocado, mixed greens and tomato slices on each tortilla.

Season with salt and pepper.

Roll up the tortillas tightly and cut in half.

Preparation Time: 10 minutes

Benefits: Offers a good balance of protein from turkey and healthy fats from avocado, aiding in muscle recovery and providing sustained energy. The whole wheat tortillas add fiber for digestive health.

Grilled Chicken and Vegetable Bowl

For: 2 people

Ingredients:

2 chicken breasts

1 zucchini, sliced

1 bell pepper, sliced

1/2 red onion, sliced

2 cups brown rice, cooked

2 tablespoons olive oil

Salt and pepper to taste

Preparation:

Preheat the grill to medium-high heat.

Brush chicken and vegetables with olive oil and season with salt and pepper.

Grill the chicken for about 6-7 minutes per side or until fully cooked.

Grill vegetables until tender and slightly charred.

Slice the chicken and serve on top of cooked brown rice along with grilled vegetables.

Preparation Time: 25 minutes

Benefits: Chicken provides high-quality protein for muscle maintenance. Brown rice is a good source of complex carbohydrates for energy, grilled vegetables add fiber and essential nutrients.

Lentil Soup with Spinach

For: 2 people

Ingredients:

1 cup dried lentils

4 cups vegetable broth

1 cup fresh spinach leaves

1 carrot, diced

1 onion, diced

2 cloves garlic, minced

1 teaspoon cumin

Salt and pepper to taste

Preparation:

In a large pot, sauté onion, carrot and garlic until soft.

Add lentils, vegetable broth and cumin.

Bring to a boil then reduce heat to simmer for about 20 minutes until lentils are tender.

Stir in spinach and cook until wilted.

Preparation Time: 30 minutes

Benefits: Lentils are an excellent source of protein and fiber, supporting muscle health and digestive well-being. Spinach provides iron and folate, which are essential for energy production.

Tofu Stir-Fry with Broccoli and Peppers

For: 2 people

Ingredients:

1 block tofu, pressed and cubed

2 cups broccoli florets

1 red bell pepper, sliced

1 tablespoon soy sauce

1 tablespoon sesame oil

2 cloves garlic, minced

1 teaspoon grated ginger

Preparation:

Heat sesame oil in a large skillet or wok over medium-high heat.

Add garlic and ginger, and sauté for about 1 minute until fragrant.

Add the tofu cubes and cook until golden brown on all sides.

Add broccoli and bell pepper, and stir-fry for about 5 minutes until the vegetables are tender-crisp.

Drizzle soy sauce over the mixture and stir to coat evenly.

Preparation Time: 20 minutes

Benefits: Tofu is a great source of plant-based protein, essential for muscle repair and growth. Broccoli and bell peppers are packed with vitamins C and K, promoting immune health and bone strength.

Snack Recipes

Almond and Date Energy Balls

For: 2 people

Ingredients:

1 cup Medjool dates, pitted

1/2 cup raw almonds

1/4 cup shredded coconut

1 tablespoon chia seeds

Preparation:

In a food processor, blend the almonds until finely chopped.

Add dates and chia seeds to the almonds and process until the mixture forms a sticky dough.

Roll the mixture into small balls then roll each ball in shredded coconut until evenly coated.

Refrigerate for at least 30 minutes before serving.

Preparation Time: 15 minutes

Benefits: These energy balls are rich in healthy fats and protein from almonds and natural sugars from dates, providing a quick energy boost. Chia seeds add fiber and omega-3 fatty acids, supporting heart health.

Greek Yogurt and Mixed Berries

For: 2 people

Ingredients:

1 cup Greek yogurt

1 cup mixed berries (blueberries, strawberries, raspberries)

2 teaspoons honey

A sprinkle of granola (optional)

Preparation:

Divide the Greek yogurt into two bowls.

Top each bowl with mixed berries and a drizzle of honey.

Add a sprinkle of granola for added texture if desired.

Preparation Time: 5 minutes

Benefits: Greek yogurt provides a high-protein base, aiding muscle recovery. Berries offer antioxidants that help reduce inflammation and oxidative stress.

Cucumber and Hummus Plates

For: 2 people

Ingredients:

1 large cucumber, sliced

1 cup hummus

Paprika for garnish

Preparation:

Arrange cucumber slices on a plate.

Place a bowl of hummus in the center.

Sprinkle hummus with a bit of paprika for flavor and color.

Preparation Time: 10 minutes

Benefits: Cucumber is hydrating and low in calories, while hummus provides a good mix of protein and fiber, making this a filling yet light snack.

Avocado Toast with Cherry Tomatoes

For: 2 people

Ingredients:

2 slices of whole-grain bread

1 ripe avocado

1/2 cup cherry tomatoes, halved

Salt and pepper to taste

Red pepper flakes (optional)

Preparation:

Toast the bread slices.

Mash the avocado and spread it evenly on each slice of toast.

Top with halved cherry tomatoes.

Season with salt, pepper and red pepper flakes if desired.

Preparation Time: 10 minutes

Benefits: Avocado provides healthy fats that are essential for joint health and skin elasticity. Whole grain bread offers fiber for digestion and tomatoes are rich in vitamins and antioxidants.

Apple Slices with Peanut Butter and Granola

For: 2 people

Ingredients:

1 large apple, sliced

1/4 cup natural peanut butter

1/4 cup granola

Preparation:

Slice the apple into thin wedges.

Spread peanut butter on each apple slice.

Sprinkle granola over the peanut butter for a crunchy texture.

Preparation Time: 5 minutes

Benefits: Apples provide a natural sweetness and fiber, while peanut butter adds protein and healthy fats. Granola adds a satisfying crunch and extra fiber, making this a balanced snack for sustained energy.

Dinner Recipes

Salmon with Asparagus and Quinoa

For: 2 people

Ingredients:

2 salmon fillets (about 6 oz each)

1 bunch of asparagus, trimmed

1 cup quinoa

2 tablespoons olive oil

Lemon wedges for serving

Salt and pepper to taste

Preparation:

Preheat the oven to 400°F (200°C).

Place the salmon and asparagus on a baking sheet, drizzle with olive oil and season with salt and pepper.

Roast in the oven for about 15-20 minutes until the salmon is cooked through and the asparagus is tender.

Meanwhile, cook quinoa according to package instructions.

Serve the salmon and asparagus with cooked quinoa and a wedge of lemon.

Preparation Time: 30 minutes

Benefits: Salmon is rich in omega-3 fatty acids, which are great for heart health and reducing inflammation. Quinoa provides a gluten-free source of protein and fiber, supporting muscle repair and digestive health.

Beef and Vegetable Kabobs

For: 2 people

Ingredients:

1 lb beef, cut into cubes

1 zucchini, sliced into rounds

1 yellow bell pepper, cut into chunks

1 red onion, cut into chunks

2 tablespoons olive oil

Salt and pepper to taste

Preparation:

Preheat your grill to medium-high heat.

Thread beef, zucchini, bell pepper and onion onto skewers.

Brush the kabobs with olive oil and season with salt and pepper.

Grill for about 10-15 minutes, turning occasionally, until the beef is cooked to your liking and vegetables are charred and tender.

Preparation Time: 30 minutes

Benefits: Beef provides high-quality protein and iron, which are vital for muscle health and energy levels. Vegetables add fiber and essential nutrients.

Spinach and Ricotta Stuffed Portobello Mushrooms

For: 2 people

Ingredients:

4 large Portobello mushroom caps, stems and gills removed

1 cup ricotta cheese

1 cup spinach, chopped

1/4 cup grated Parmesan cheese

2 cloves garlic, minced

2 tablespoons olive oil

Salt and pepper to taste

Preparation:

Preheat the oven to 375°F (190°C).

In a bowl, mix ricotta, spinach, Parmesan, garlic, salt and pepper.

Place mushroom caps on a baking sheet and brush with olive oil.

Stuff each mushroom with the ricotta mixture.

Bake for about 20 minutes, until the mushrooms are tender and the filling is hot.

Preparation Time: 30 minutes

Benefits: Portobello mushrooms are low in calories but high in fiber and protein. Ricotta and spinach provide calcium and iron, essential for bone health and muscle function.

Lemon Herb Tilapia with Sweet Potatoes

For: 2 people

Ingredients:

2 tilapia fillets (about 6 oz each)

2 small sweet potatoes, peeled and diced

2 tablespoons olive oil

1 lemon, juiced and zested

2 teaspoons dried herbs (thyme, oregano, or basil)

Salt and pepper to taste

Preparation:

Preheat the oven to 400°F (200°C).

Toss the diced sweet potatoes in 1 tablespoon of olive oil, salt and pepper. Spread them on a baking sheet and roast in the oven for about 25 minutes until tender and golden.

Meanwhile, mix lemon juice, zest, herbs and the remaining olive oil in a small bowl. Season the tilapia fillets with salt and pepper then brush them with the lemon herb mixture.

In the last 10 minutes of cooking the sweet potatoes, add the tilapia fillets to the baking sheet.

Bake until the fish is flaky and cooked through for about 10 minutes.

Preparation Time: 35 minutes

Benefits: Tilapia is a lean source of protein that helps in muscle repair and building. Sweet potatoes are a rich source of vitamin A and fiber which promote skin health and digestive well-being.

Pre-Workout Recipes

Oatmeal with Banana and Chia Seeds

For: 2 people

Preparation Time: 10 minutes

Ingredients:

1 cup rolled oats

2 cups water or milk

1 banana, sliced

2 tablespoons chia seeds

1 tablespoon honey or maple syrup

Preparation:

Cook the oats in water or milk according to package instructions.

Once cooked, stir in chia seeds and sweeten with honey or maple syrup.

Top with banana slices.

Serve warm.

Benefits: Oats provide a steady supply of carbohydrates for energy. Chia seeds are rich in omega- 3 fatty acids which help maintain cell membrane health and reduce inflammation. Bananas are a great source of potassium which helps in muscle function and prevents cramping.

Greek Yogurt with Mixed Nuts and Berries

For: 2 people

Preparation Time: 5 minutes

Ingredients:

2 cups Greek yogurt

1/2 cup mixed berries (blueberries, raspberries, strawberries)

1/4 cup mixed nuts (almonds, walnuts), chopped

Preparation:

Divide the yogurt into two bowls.

Top each bowl with berries and chopped nuts.

Benefits: Greek yogurt provides a high-quality protein to support muscle synthesis. Berries offer antioxidants to combat oxidative stress and nuts provide healthy fats for sustained energy.

Smoothie with Spinach, Mango, and Flaxseed

For: 2 people

Preparation Time: 5 minutes

Ingredients:

1 cup fresh spinach

1 mango, peeled and chopped

1 tablespoon flaxseed

1 cup almond milk or water

Ice cubes (optional)

Preparation:

Blend all ingredients in a blender until smooth.

Serve chilled.

Benefits: Spinach is rich in iron which is crucial for energy production. Mango provides quick- releasing sugars for an energy boost. Flaxseeds are a good source of fiber and omega-3 fatty acids which help in sustained energy release.

Avocado Toast with Egg

For: 2 people

Preparation Time: 10 minutes

Ingredients:

2 slices whole-grain bread

1 avocado

2 eggs

Salt and pepper to taste

Preparation:

Toast the bread slices.

Mash the avocado and spread evenly on each slice of toast.

Fry or poach the eggs and place one on top of each avocado toast.

Season with salt and pepper.

Serve immediately.

Benefits: Avocado provides healthy fats for a slow and steady energy release. Eggs are a great source of protein and choline which helps in muscle control and energy levels. Whole-grain bread offers complex carbohydrates for sustained energy.

Peanut Butter and Jelly Energy Balls

For: 2 people

Preparation Time: 15 minutes (plus chilling)

Ingredients:

1 cup oats

1/2 cup natural peanut butter

1/4 cup jelly or jam of choice

1/4 cup ground flaxseed

Preparation:

In a bowl, mix all ingredients until well combined.

Roll the mixture into small balls.

Place in the refrigerator to chill for at least 1 hour before serving.

Benefits: Peanut butter provides a good source of protein and healthy fats. Oats and flaxseed supply fiber and slow-releasing energy. The jelly adds a quick burst of energy due to its simple sugars.

Post Workout Recipes

Grilled Chicken and Avocado Salad

For: 2 people

Preparation Time: 20 minutes

Ingredients:

2 chicken breasts

1 ripe avocado, sliced

4 cups mixed greens (spinach, arugula, and romaine)

1/2 cucumber, sliced

10 cherry tomatoes, halved

2 tablespoons olive oil

1 tablespoon balsamic vinegar

Salt and pepper to taste

Preparation:

Grill the chicken breasts until fully cooked and slice them.

In a large bowl, combine mixed greens, cucumber, cherry tomatoes and avocado.

Add the sliced chicken to the salad.

Drizzle with olive oil and balsamic vinegar then season with salt and pepper.

Toss everything together and serve.

Benefits: Provides lean protein from chicken for muscle repair, healthy fats from avocado for recovery and antioxidants from fresh vegetables to reduce inflammation.

Quinoa and Black Bean Bowl

For: 2 people

Preparation Time: 30 minutes

Ingredients:

1 cup quinoa

1 can black beans, drained and rinsed

1 red bell pepper, diced

1/2 red onion, diced

1 cup corn kernels

2 tablespoons lime juice

1 teaspoon cumin

Fresh cilantro, chopped

Salt and pepper to taste

Preparation:

Cook quinoa according to package instructions.

In a large bowl, mix cooked quinoa, black beans, bell pepper, onion and corn.

Add lime juice, cumin, cilantro, salt and pepper. Stir to combine.

Serve warm or at room temperature.

Benefits: Rich in plant-based protein and fiber from quinoa and black beans which aid in muscle recovery and provide sustained energy. The fresh veggies contribute essential vitamins and minerals.

Turkey and Sweet Potato Skillet

For: 2 people

Preparation Time: 45 minutes

Ingredients:

1 lb ground turkey

2 medium sweet potatoes, diced

1 green bell pepper, diced

1 onion, diced

2 cloves garlic, minced

1 tablespoon olive oil

1 teaspoon smoked paprika

Salt and pepper to taste

Preparation:

Heat olive oil in a large skillet over medium heat.

Add garlic and onion, sauté until translucent.

Add ground turkey and cook until browned.

Stir in sweet potatoes, bell pepper, smoked paprika, salt and pepper.

Cover and cook until sweet potatoes are tender.

Serve hot.

Benefits: Turkey provides high-quality protein for muscle repair, while sweet potatoes offer complex carbohydrates for replenishing glycogen stores. Bell peppers and onions provide antioxidants and vitamins.

Salmon with Steamed Broccoli and Almonds

For: 2 people

Preparation Time: 25 minutes

Ingredients:

2 salmon fillets (about 6 oz each)

2 cups broccoli florets

1/4 cup sliced almonds

2 tablespoons olive oil

Lemon wedges for serving

Salt and pepper to taste

Preparation:

Preheat the oven to 400°F (200°C).

Place salmon fillets on a baking sheet, drizzle with 1 tablespoon olive oil and season with salt and pepper.

Roast in the oven for about 15-20 minutes, until cooked through.

Steam broccoli until tender then toss with remaining olive oil and sliced almonds.

Serve salmon with steamed almond broccoli and a wedge of lemon.

Benefits: Salmon is rich in omega-3 fatty acids, essential for reducing inflammation and aiding recovery. Broccoli and almonds provide fiber, vitamins and additional healthy fats.

Greek Yogurt with Berries and Honey

For: 2 people

Preparation Time: 10 minutes

Ingredients:

2 cups Greek yogurt

1 cup mixed berries (strawberries, blueberries, raspberries)

2 tablespoons honey

1/4 cup granola (optional)

Preparation:

Divide the Greek yogurt between two bowls.

Top each bowl with half of the mixed berries and a tablespoon of honey.

Sprinkle granola on top if desired for added texture.

Benefits: Greek yogurt is a great source of protein, crucial for muscle repair post-workout. Berries add antioxidants for reducing exercise-induced oxidative stress and honey provides a gentle sweetness and quick energy replenishment.

CHAPTER 9

31 DAYS MEAL PLAN

Day 1:

Breakfast: Banana and Almond Butter Toast

Lunch: Quinoa Chickpea Salad

Snack: Almond and Date Energy Balls

Dinner: Salmon with Asparagus and Quinoa

Day 2:

Breakfast: Greek Yogurt Parfait with Mixed Berries and Granola

Lunch: Turkey and Avocado Wrap

Snack: Greek Yogurt and Mixed Berries

Dinner: Chicken Stir-Fry with Broccoli and Bell Peppers

Day 3:

Breakfast: Spinach and Mushroom Omelette

Lunch: Grilled Chicken and Vegetable Bowl

Snack: Cucumber and Hummus Plates

Dinner: Beef and Vegetable Kabobs

Day 4:

Breakfast: Avocado and Egg Breakfast Salad

Lunch: Lentil Soup with Spinach

Snack: Avocado Toast with Cherry Tomatoes

Dinner: Spinach and Ricotta Stuffed Portobello Mushrooms

Day 5:

Breakfast: Blueberry and Walnut Oatmeal

Lunch: Tofu Stir-Fry with Broccoli and Peppers

Snack: Apple Slices with Peanut Butter and Granola

Dinner: Lemon Herb Tilapia with Sweet Potatoes

Day 6:

Breakfast: Banana and Almond Butter Toast

Lunch: Turkey and Avocado Wrap

Snack: Greek Yogurt and Mixed Berries

Dinner: Chicken Stir-Fry with Broccoli and Bell Peppers

Day 7:

Breakfast: Greek Yogurt Parfait with Mixed Berries and Granola

Lunch: Grilled Chicken and Vegetable Bowl

Snack: Almond and Date Energy Balls

Dinner: Salmon with Asparagus and Quinoa

Day 8:

Breakfast: Spinach and Mushroom Omelette

Lunch: Lentil Soup with Spinach

Snack: Cucumber and Hummus Plates

Dinner: Beef and Vegetable Kabobs

Day 9:

Breakfast: Avocado and Egg Breakfast Salad

Lunch: Quinoa Chickpea Salad

Snack: Apple Slices with Peanut Butter and Granola

Dinner: Lemon Herb Tilapia with Sweet Potatoes

Day 10:

Breakfast: Blueberry and Walnut Oatmeal

Lunch: Tofu Stir-Fry with Broccoli and Peppers

Snack: Avocado Toast with Cherry Tomatoes

Dinner: Spinach and Ricotta Stuffed Portobello Mushrooms

Day 11:

Breakfast: Spinach and Mushroom Omelette

Lunch: Turkey and Avocado Wrap

Snack: Almond and Date Energy Balls

Dinner: Chicken Stir-Fry with Broccoli and Bell Peppers

Day 12:

Breakfast: Avocado and Egg Breakfast Salad

Lunch: Grilled Chicken and Vegetable Bowl

Snack: Cucumber and Hummus Plates

Dinner: Beef and Vegetable Kabobs

Day 13:

Breakfast: Blueberry and Walnut Oatmeal

Lunch: Lentil Soup with Spinach

Snack: Apple Slices with Peanut Butter and Granola

Dinner: Spinach and Ricotta Stuffed Portobello Mushrooms

Day 14:

Breakfast: Banana and Almond Butter Toast

Lunch: Tofu Stir-Fry with Broccoli and Peppers

Snack: Greek Yogurt and Mixed Berries

Dinner: Lemon Herb Tilapia with Sweet Potatoes

Day 15:

Breakfast: Greek Yogurt Parfait with Mixed Berries and Granola

Lunch: Quinoa Chickpea Salad

Snack: Avocado Toast with Cherry Tomatoes

Dinner: Salmon with Asparagus and Quinoa

Day 16:

Breakfast: Spinach and Mushroom Omelette

Lunch: Turkey and Avocado Wrap

Snack: Cucumber and Hummus Plates

Dinner: Chicken Stir-Fry with Broccoli and Bell Peppers

Day 17:

Breakfast: Avocado and Egg Breakfast Salad

Lunch: Grilled Chicken and Vegetable Bowl

Snack: Apple Slices with Peanut Butter and Granola

Dinner: Beef and Vegetable Kabobs

Day 18:

Breakfast: Blueberry and Walnut Oatmeal

Lunch: Lentil Soup with Spinach

Snack: Greek Yogurt and Mixed Berries

Dinner: Spinach and Ricotta Stuffed Portobello Mushrooms

Day 19:

Breakfast: Banana and Almond Butter Toast

Lunch: Tofu Stir-Fry with Broccoli and Peppers

Snack: Almond and Date Energy Balls

Dinner: Lemon Herb Tilapia with Sweet Potatoes

Day 20:

Breakfast: Greek Yogurt Parfait with Mixed Berries and Granola

Lunch: Quinoa Chickpea Salad

Snack: Avocado Toast with Cherry Tomatoes

Dinner: Salmon with Asparagus and Quinoa

Day 21:

Breakfast: Spinach and Mushroom Omelette

Lunch: Turkey and Avocado Wrap

Snack: Cucumber and Hummus Plates

Dinner: Chicken Stir-Fry with Broccoli and Bell Peppers

Day 22:

Breakfast: Avocado and Egg Breakfast Salad

Lunch: Grilled Chicken and Vegetable Bowl

Snack: Apple Slices with Peanut Butter and Granola

Dinner: Beef and Vegetable Kabobs

Day 23:

Breakfast: Blueberry and Walnut Oatmeal

Lunch: Lentil Soup with Spinach

Snack: Greek Yogurt and Mixed Berries

Dinner: Spinach and Ricotta Stuffed Portobello Mushrooms

Day 24:

Breakfast: Banana and Almond Butter Toast

Lunch: Tofu Stir-Fry with Broccoli and Peppers

Snack: Almond and Date Energy Balls

Dinner: Lemon Herb Tilapia with Sweet Potatoes

Day 25:

Breakfast: Greek Yogurt Parfait with Mixed Berries and Granola

Lunch: Quinoa Chickpea Salad

Snack: Avocado Toast with Cherry Tomatoes

Dinner: Salmon with Asparagus and Quinoa

Day 26:

Breakfast: Spinach and Mushroom Omelette

Lunch: Turkey and Avocado Wrap

Snack: Cucumber and Hummus Plates

Dinner: Chicken Stir-Fry with Broccoli and Bell Peppers

Day 27:

Breakfast: Avocado and Egg Breakfast Salad

Lunch: Grilled Chicken and Vegetable Bowl

Snack: Apple Slices with Peanut Butter and Granola

Dinner: Beef and Vegetable Kabobs

Day 28:

Breakfast: Blueberry and Walnut Oatmeal

Lunch: Lentil Soup with Spinach

Snack: Greek Yogurt and Mixed Berries

Dinner: Spinach and Ricotta Stuffed Portobello Mushrooms

Day 29:

Breakfast: Banana and Almond Butter Toast

Lunch: Tofu Stir-Fry with Broccoli and Peppers

Snack: Almond and Date Energy Balls

Dinner: Lemon Herb Tilapia with Sweet Potatoes

Day 30:

Breakfast: Greek Yogurt Parfait with Mixed Berries and Granola

Lunch: Quinoa Chickpea Salad

Snack: Avocado Toast with Cherry Tomatoes

Dinner: Salmon with Asparagus and Quinoa

Day 31:

Breakfast: Spinach and Mushroom Omelette

Lunch: Turkey and Avocado Wrap

Snack: Cucumber and Hummus Plates

Dinner: Chicken Stir-Fry with Broccoli and Bell Peppers

CHAPTER 10

WALL PILATES WORKOUT PLAN FOR BEGINNERS

Day 1: Getting Started

- Wall Push-Aways (3 sets of 10)
- Wall Slides (3 sets of 10)
- Wall-Assisted Leg Swings (10 swings each leg)
- Wall Toe Taps (3 sets of 10 on each leg)

Day 2: Core Introduction

- Wall Mountain Climbers (3 sets of 15)
- Wall Plank (hold for 20 seconds, repeat 3 times)

Day 3: Upper Body Basics

- Wall Push-Ups (3 sets of 8)
- Wall Angels (3 sets of 10)
- Wall Chest Squeeze (hold for 5 seconds, repeat 10 times)

Day 4: Lower Body Activation

- Wall Squats (3 sets of 10)
- Wall Assisted Lunges (3 sets of 8 each leg)
- Wall Calf Raises (3 sets of 15)

Day 5: Flexibility Foundations

- Wall Hamstring Stretch (hold for 30 seconds each leg)
- Wall Supported Chest Opener (hold for 30 seconds)
- Wall Angel (3 sets of 10)

Day 6: Full Body Integration

- Wall Push-Ups (3 sets of 8)
- Wall Squats (3 sets of 10)
- Standing Wall Leg Lifts (3 sets of 10 each leg)

Day 7: BREAKING

Day 8: Core Enhancement

- Wall Mountain Climbers (3 sets of 20)
- Wall Plank (hold for 30 seconds, repeat 3 times)

Day 9: Upper Body Strength

- Wall Push-Ups (3 sets of 10)
- Wall Bicep Curls (using a resistance band, 3 sets of 10)
- Wall Angels (3 sets of 12)

Day 10: Lower Body Focus

- Wall Glute Bridges (3 sets of 12)
- Wall Side Leg Lifts (3 sets of 10 each side)
- Wall Assisted Lunges (3 sets of 10 each leg)

Day 11: Balance and Flexibility

- Wall Supported Warrior Pose (hold for 20 seconds each side)
- Wall-to-Floor Reach (3 sets of 10)
- Wall Supported Tree Pose (hold for 15 seconds each side)

Day 12: Full Body Coordination

- Wall Pelvic Tilts (3 sets of 15)
- Wall Squats (3 sets of 12)
- Wall Push-Ups with one leg raised (3 sets of 6 each leg)

Day 13: Core Reinforcement

- Wall Mountain Climbers (3 sets of 25)
- Wall Plank with leg lift (3 sets of 5 lifts each leg)

Day 14: BREAKING

-

Day 15: Upper Body Endurance

- Wall Tricep Dips (using a chair, 3 sets of 8)
- Wall Chest Squeeze (hold for 10 seconds, repeat 10 times)

- Wall Angels (3 sets of 15)

Day 16: Lower Body Strength

- Wall Squats (3 sets of 15)
- Wall Calf Raises (3 sets of 20)
- Wall Glute Bridges (3 sets of 15)

Day 17: Flexibility Day

- Wall Hamstring Stretch (hold for 40 seconds each leg)
- Wall Butterfly Stretch (sit against the wall, press knees down and hold for 30 seconds)
- Wall Supported Forward Bend (hold for 30 seconds)

Day 18: Full Body Challenge

- Wall Push-Ups (3 sets of 12)
- Wall Squats with toe lift at the top (3 sets of 12)
- Standing Wall Leg Lifts with a hold at the top (hold 5 seconds, 10 times each leg)

Day 19: Core Stability

- Wall Plank with alternating knee taps (3 sets of 30 seconds)
- Wall Mountain Climbers (3 sets of 20 with a slower, controlled motion)

Day 20: Upper Body and Core

- Wall Push-Ups with alternating shoulder taps (3 sets of 10)
- Wall Slides with a pause at bottom (3 sets of 10, hold bottom for 5 seconds)
- Wall Chest Squeeze with a slow release (3 sets of 10, squeeze for 5 seconds, release slowly)

Day 21: BREAKING

Day 22: Lower Body Power

- Wall Sit (hold for 30 seconds, repeat 3 times)
- Wall Assisted Pistol Squats (3 sets of 5 each leg, use wall for balance)
- Wall Calf Raises with a pause at the top (3 sets of 15, hold top for 3 seconds)

Day 23: Flexibility and Mobility

- Wall Supported Full Body Stretch (stand facing away from wall, reach overhead and lean back against wall, hold for 30 seconds)

- Wall Supported Pigeon Pose (each leg, hold for 30 seconds)
- Wall Angel with a focus on deep breathing (3 sets of 12, breathe in on rise, out on lower)

Day 24: Full Body Endurance

- Wall Push-Ups (3 sets of 15)
- Wall Squats with a single leg raise at the top (3 sets of 10 each leg)
- Standing Wall Leg Lifts with a pulse at the top (3 sets of 10 each leg, pulse 3 times)

Day 25: Core and Lower Body Synthesis

- Wall Plank with leg raises (3 sets of 10 each leg)
- Wall Mountain Climbers with a twist towards opposite elbow (3 sets of 15 each side)

Day 26: Upper Body Resilience

- Wall Push-Ups with a wide hand placement (3 sets of 10)
- Wall Tricep Dips (using a chair, 3 sets of 10)
- Wall Bicep Curls with a slower motion (using a resistance band, 3 sets of 10, go slow up and down)

Day 27: Lower Body and Balance

- Wall Supported Single Leg Squat (3 sets of 8 each leg)
- Wall Assisted Lunges with a back leg lift (3 sets of 10 each leg)
- Wall Calf Raises on one leg (3 sets of 10 each leg)

Day 28: BREAKING

Day 29: Flexibility Focus

- Wall Hamstring Stretch with deeper reach (each leg, hold for 40 seconds)
- Wall Supported Chest Opener with arms wider (hold for 40 seconds)
- Wall Supported Downward Dog (hold for 40 seconds)

Day 30: Full Body Review

- Combine favorite exercises from previous days:
- Wall Push-Ups
- Wall Plank
- Wall Squats
- Wall Angels

- Wall Mountain Climbers

Perform each exercise for 3 sets of 10-15 reps or 30 seconds each.

CHAPTER 11

INTERMEDIATE TO ADVANCED WALL PILATES WORKOUT PLAN

Day 1: Review and Prep

- Review fundamental techniques and ensure form is perfected in basic exercises.

Day 2: Intermediate Core Exercises

- Wall Bridges (3 sets of 12)
- Wall Oblique Twists (3 sets of 10 each side)

Day 3: Intermediate Upper Body Strength

- Wall Plank Shoulder Taps (3 sets of 10 each side)
- Wall Tricep Dips (using a chair, 3 sets of 10)
- Incline Wall Push-Ups (3 sets of 12)

Day 4: Intermediate Lower Body and Glutes

- Wall Pistol Squats (3 sets of 8 each leg)
- Elevated Wall Glute Bridge (3 sets of 12)
- Wall Lateral Slide Squats (3 sets of 10 each direction)

Day 5: Enhancing Flexibility and Balance

- Wall Supported Warrior Pose (Hold for 30 seconds each side)
- Wall Angel (3 sets of 12)

Day 6: Full Body Intermediate Workouts

- Wall Mountain Climbers (3 sets of 15)
- Side Wall Plank (Hold for 20 seconds, 3 sets each side)
- Wall Push-Up with Leg Lift (3 sets of 10)

Day 7: Rest and Active Recovery

- Light stretching and flexibility work focusing on the Wall Supported Chest Opener and Wall Hamstring Stretch.

Day 8: Advanced Core Challenges

- Wall V-Sits (3 sets of 10)
- Wall Leg Raises with a Twist (3 sets of 10 each side)

Day 9: Advanced Upper Body Power

- Elevated Wall Handstand Push-Ups (3 sets of 8)
- Wall Climbs (3 sets of 5 each side)
- Dynamic Wall Chest Flies (3 sets of 10)

Day 10: Advanced Lower Body Dynamics

- One-Legged Wall Squat (3 sets of 8 each leg)
- Wall Supported Warrior III (Hold for 20 seconds each leg)

Day 11: Pushing Flexibility Limits

- Vertical Wall Splits (Hold for 30 seconds)
- Wall Supported Downward Dog (Hold for 40 seconds)

Day 12: Full Body Advanced Workouts

- Wall Plank with Leg Thread (3 sets of 10 each leg)
- Wall Reverse Plank (Hold for 30 seconds, 3 sets)
- Vertical Wall Run (3 sets of 20 seconds)

Day 13: Integration of Skills

- Combine selected exercises from intermediate and advanced routines that focus on strength, flexibility and balance.

Day 14: Rest and Reflect

- Assess progress, adjust goals and prepare for continued practice.

Day 15: Core Mastery

- Wall Plank Rotations (3 sets of 10 each side)
- One-Arm Wall Push (3 sets of 8 each arm)

Day 16: Upper Body Refinement

- Wall Reverse Flys (3 sets of 12)
- Wall Mounted Pike Press (3 sets of 10)

Day 17: Lower Body Precision

- Wall Split Squat Jumps (3 sets of 10 each leg)
- Diagonal Wall Squat (3 sets of 10 each direction)

Day 18: Flexibility Deep Dive

- Wall Supported Warrior Pose (Hold for 40 seconds, repeat 3 times each side)
- Wall Butterfly Stretch (Hold for 30 seconds, 3 sets)

Day 19: Advanced Full Body Integration

- One-Legged Wall Squat (3 sets of 8 each leg)
- Wall Plank with Leg Thread (3 sets of 10 each leg)
- Wall Reverse Plank (Hold for 35 seconds, 3 sets)

Day 20: Active Recovery and Mindfulness

- Wall Slide Breathing (5 minutes of focused breathing)
- Gentle stretching using Wall Hamstring Stretch and Wall Supported Forward Bend

Day 21: Rest and Reflect

- Review progress, journal experiences, and adjust for personal growth and challenges.

Day 22: High-Intensity Core

- Wall V-Sits (4 sets of 12)
- Wall Leg Raises with a Twist (4 sets of 12 each side)

Day 23: Upper Body Endurance

- Dynamic Wall Chest Flies (4 sets of 12)
- Wall Climbs (3 sets of 6 each side)

Day 24: Lower Body Endurance

- Wall Supported Warrior III (Hold for 30 seconds, 4 sets each leg)
- Wall Lateral Slide Squats (4 sets of 12 each direction)

Day 25: Flexibility and Balance

- Vertical Wall Splits (Hold for 40 seconds)
- Wall-Assisted Downward Dog (Hold for 45 seconds)

Day 26: Full Body Challenge

- Wall-Assisted Handstand Push-Ups (3 sets of 10)
- Wall Reverse Plank (Hold for 40 seconds, 3 sets)
- Vertical Wall Run (4 sets of 25 seconds)

Day 27: Dynamic Strength and Coordination

- Wall Assisted One-Arm Push-Ups (3 sets of 8 each arm)
- Wall Plank Knee to Elbow (3 sets of 12 each side)
- Wall Jump Squats (3 sets of 10)

Day 28: Endurance and Stability

- Extended Wall Sit (Hold for 60 seconds, 3 sets)
- Wall Supported Single-Leg Deadlift (3 sets of 10 each leg)
- Wall Slide Lunges (3 sets of 12 each leg)

Day 29: Flexibility and Core Focus

- Wall Supported Pike Stretch (Hold for 40 seconds, 3 sets)
- Wall Hanging Leg Raises (3 sets of 10)
- Wall Twisting Planks (3 sets of 10 each side)

Day 30: Full Body Integration and Flow

- Wall Handstand (Hold for 20 seconds, 3 attempts)
- Wall T-Push-Ups (3 sets of 10 each side)
- Wall Supported Warrior III to Single Leg Squat (3 sets of 6 each leg)

9 BONUSES

Audiobook

The audiobook included with "Wall Pilates Workouts for Women" is a valuable resource for those who have busy schedules and need to optimize their time. With the audiobook, you can listen to detailed instructions and insights about Pilates exercises and techniques while commuting, doing household chores or during any other activity where reading a physical book isn't convenient. This flexibility allows you to absorb the material and understand the nuances of each exercise which can significantly improve your practice. Additionally, having audio guidance can help you focus on performing the exercises correctly, minimizing the risk of injury, and ensuring you get the most out of your workout.

Music for Pilates

Music specially curated for Pilates can greatly enhance your workout experience by creating an environment that is both motivating and calming. The right music can help you maintain a steady pace, synchronize your movements and stay focused throughout your exercises. This can be particularly beneficial for maintaining the rhythm and flow essential in Pilates, leading to better coordination and fluidity in your movements. Moreover, enjoyable music can make your workouts more pleasant and less of a chore. Thus, encouraging you to stick to your routine and achieve your fitness goals.

Ebook – Mindfulness Meditation

The mindfulness meditation ebook is a perfect complement to your physical Pilates practice, offering mental and emotional benefits that can enhance your overall well-being. Understanding and practicing mindfulness can help reduce stress, improve mental clarity and increase your awareness of your body and breath. All of which are crucial for maximizing the benefits of Pilates. By integrating mindfulness into your routine, you can improve your concentration and presence during exercises, leading to more effective workouts and a deeper connection to your body. This holistic approach can help you achieve a balanced mind-body connection, essential for overall health and fitness.

Food Calorie Calculator

The food calorie calculator is an essential tool for anyone looking to optimize their diet and achieve specific fitness goals. By accurately tracking your daily caloric intake, you can ensure that you are consuming the right amount of calories to fuel your body for Pilates workouts while also managing your weight. This tool can help you make informed dietary choices, balancing your energy intake with your expenditure to support muscle toning and overall body transformation. With precise calorie tracking, you can tailor your nutrition plan to fit your individual needs, enhancing the effectiveness of your exercise regimen.

Full Macro Calculator

The full macro calculator takes your nutritional planning to the next level by helping you balance your intake of proteins, carbohydrates and fats. Proper macronutrient distribution is crucial for optimizing your performance and results in Pilates. For example, adequate protein intake supports muscle repair and growth, while the right balance of carbs and fats provides sustained energy for your workouts. By using the macro calculator, you can customize your diet to meet your specific fitness goals, whether they are building strength, increasing flexibility or toning your body. This personalized approach to nutrition ensures that you are fueling your body correctly to maximize the benefits of your Pilates practice.

Ebook - Intermittent Fasting for Women over 50

The guide to intermittent fasting for women over 50 offers tailored nutritional strategies that can enhance your metabolism and overall health, especially when combined with your Pilates routine. Intermittent fasting can help manage weight, improve insulin sensitivity and boost energy levels, making your workouts more effective and sustainable. This guide provides practical advice and tips on how to implement fasting safely and effectively, considering the unique metabolic and hormonal changes that occur with age. By integrating intermittent fasting into your lifestyle, you can support your fitness goals and enhance your overall well-being.

Printable – Fitness Planner

The printable fitness planner is an invaluable tool for organizing and tracking your Pilates workouts, helping you stay motivated and consistent. With this planner, you can set clear goals, schedule your exercises and monitor your progress over time. Keeping a detailed record of your workouts can help you identify patterns, celebrate achievements and stay accountable to your fitness journey. This structured approach can make it easier to maintain a regular exercise routine, ultimately leading to better results and a more disciplined approach to your health and fitness.

Printable – Shopping List

The printable shopping list is designed to make your grocery shopping more efficient and aligned with your fitness goals. By planning your meals and creating a shopping list, you can ensure that you have all the necessary ingredients for a nutritious diet that supports your Pilates practice. This list can help you make healthier food choices, avoid impulse purchases and stick to a balanced diet that provides the energy and nutrients needed for effective workouts. Having a well-organized shopping list can simplify meal preparation and ensure that you stay on track with your dietary and fitness objectives.

Video

The included videos offer a visual and practical guide to performing Pilates exercises correctly, which can be especially helpful for beginners or those looking to refine their technique.

Scan the QR CODE on the next page

Scan the QR CODE

Printed in Great Britain
by Amazon

46628553R00059